Praise for *Still Sexy After All These Years?*

"We are sexual creatures from birth to death. *Still Sexy After All These Years?* breaks new ground and explodes all the commonly accepted myths about sexuality and aging, and charts new and exciting territory."
—Christiane Northrup, M.D., author of *Mothers and Daughters,*
Women's Bodies, Women's Wisdom, and *The Wisdom of Menopause*

"Kliger and Nedelman's book is a pep talk between book covers, a warm, conversational, no-nonsense discussion of post-menopausal sexuality happily devoid of preachiness or prescriptive how-to's. Every woman over 50 can benefit from this smart, sensible, and unusually (mercifully) well-written guide."
—Letty Cottin Pogrebin, author of *Getting Over Getting Older*

We know very little about how women retain their sexual selves. This well written and inspiring book gives us insightful research on this new older woman. It clarifies expectations for the aging population and gives hope and guidelines for our sexual future. This book is a powerful contribution to sexology and a must read for baby boomers like myself, who want to believe that our sexual life can stay with us until the very end.
—Pepper Schwartz, Ph.D., author of *Everything You Know About*
Love and Sex Is Wrong and *The Gender of Sexuality*

"With its focus on diversity, *Still Sexy?* conveys more truths about women's sexual lives than a thousand so-called health news articles or a million product-pushing drug ads. As the world gets more complicated, sexually, women of every age need to know more in order to cope with the options and not be exploited."
—Leonore Tiefer, Ph.D., author of *Sex Is Not a Natural Act*

"Wise, candid, smart, and witty, the authors present truths for women over 50 about what sex for this huge group really is, and can be, all about. These two dedicated women are modern soothsayers for today's new definition of the 'sexy older woman.'"
—Patti Britton, Ph.D., author of *The Art of Sex Coaching* and president,
American Association of Sex Educators, Counselors, and Therapists
(AASECT)

"*Still Sexy After All These Years?* shows that there's plenty of light at the end of the menopause tunnel. The truth is, sexuality can be delicious for women at any age—the key is moving beyond the myths. Let this wonderful book be your passport to the rich mysteries of ongoing sexual intimacy and power."

    —Gina Ogden, Ph.D., author of *Women Who Love Sex: An Inquiry into the Expanding Spirit of Women's Erotic Experience*

"This pioneering work illuminates an unexplored territory of female sexuality, finding it lush and inhabited after all, not the barren desert of popular mythology. As always, when women tell the truth about their lives, the results are fascinating, moving, revolutionary—and the world splits open."

    —Jean Kilbourne, author of *Can't Buy My Love: How Advertising Changes the Way We Think and Feel,* creator of the *Killing Us Softly* film series, visiting research scholar, the Wellesley Centers for Women

"*Still Sexy?* illuminates the diversity in sexual desire that women experience as they age. Based on interviews and survey data with real older women throughout the U.S. Yet, its engaging style will appeal to the baby boomers who are hungry for this information as well. It is a must read for everyone who personally or professionally cares about the sexual satisfaction and well-being of older women."

    —Patricia Barthalow Koch, Ph.D., president, The Society for the Scientific Study of Sexuality and Women's Sexuality, researcher/educator

"*Still Sexy After All These Years?* raises a new concept: sexual self-esteem. It shows readers how hundreds of women have dealt with the challenges of building or rebuilding sexual self-esteem after menopause. Rich with quotes from women, *Still Sexy* introduces readers to women who've found myriad ways to be happy wherever they are with their sexuality."

    —Joani Blank, editor *Still Doing It: Women and Men over 60*

Still *Sexy* After All These Years?

The 9 Unspoken Truths About Women's Desire Beyond 50

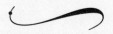

Leah Kliger, MHA,
and
Deborah Nedelman, Ph.D

A Perigee Book

Most Perigee Books are available at special quantity discounts for bulk purchases for sales promotions, premiums, fund-raising, or educational use. Special books, or book excerpts, can also be created to fit specific needs.

For details, write: Special Markets, The Berkley Publishing Group, 375 Hudson Street, New York, New York 10014.

THE BERKLEY PUBLISHING GROUP
Published by the Penguin Group
Penguin Group (USA) Inc.
375 Hudson Street, New York, New York 10014, USA
Penguin Group (Canada), 90 Eglinton Avenue East, Suite 700, Toronto, Ontario M4P 2Y3, Canada (a division of Pearson Penguin Canada Inc.)
Penguin Books Ltd., 80 Strand, London WC2R 0RL, England
Penguin Group Ireland, 25 St. Stephen's Green, Dublin 2, Ireland (a division of Penguin Books Ltd.)
Penguin Group (Australia), 250 Camberwell Road, Camberwell, Victoria 3124, Australia (a division of Pearson Australia Group Pty. Ltd.)
Penguin Books India Pvt. Ltd., 11 Community Centre, Panchsheel Park, New Delhi—110 017, India
Penguin Group (NZ), cnr. Airborne and Rosedale Roads, Albany, Auckland 1310, New Zealand (a division of Pearson New Zealand Ltd.)
Penguin Books (South Africa) (Pty.) Ltd., 24 Sturdee Avenue, Rosebank, Johannesburg 2196, South Africa

Penguin Books Ltd., Registered Offices: 80 Strand, London WC2R 0RL, England

Neither the publisher nor the authors are engaged in rendering professional advice or services to the individual reader. The ideas, procedures, and suggestions contained in this book are not intended as a substitute for consulting with your physician. All matters regarding your health require medical supervision. Neither the author nor the publisher shall be liable or responsible for any loss or damage allegedly arising from any information or suggestion in this book.

While the authors have made every effort to provide accurate telephone numbers and Internet addresses at the time of publication, neither the publisher nor the authors assume any responsibility for errors, or for changes that occur after publication. Further, publisher does not have any control over and does not assume any responsibility for author or third-party websites or their content.

PRINTING HISTORY
Perigee trade paperback edition / February 2006

PERIGEE is a registered trademark of Penguin Group (USA) Inc.
The "P" design is a trademark belonging to Penguin Group (USA) Inc.

This book has been cataloged by the Library of Congress

PRINTED IN THE UNITED STATES OF AMERICA

10 9 8 7 6 5 4 3 2 1

This book is lovingly dedicated

To our mothers, Sarah Kliger and Esther Nedelman (of blessed memory),
who filled us with womanly wisdom;

to our sisters, Robin Jollay, Susan Parcheta, and Carol Woodward,
who shared the journey;

and

to the next generations of women in our families,
Eden, Makayla, Becky, and Diana,
who inherit the legacy.

Contents

Acknowledgments

Since the inception of this project, we've been astounded at the outpouring of support, guidance, and good cheer it has generated. We would like to acknowledge and thank just a few of the thousands of people who have sustained us on our journey toward authorship.

First of all, we extend our heartfelt gratitude to our remarkably talented and articulate agent Joelle Delbourgo, who took a chance and plucked our proposal from among the hundreds on her desk, to our editor Michelle Howry, for her tireless support, editing prowess, and "can do" spirit, and to Meg Leder for shepherding our work in its later stages.

We would like to thank Carol Bloomberg, Sue Champion, Julie Clark, Tila Carrol, Judy Friedman, Sheila Guy-Snowden, Gail Jothen, Karen Kaushansky, Jan Levy, Susan Parcheta, Paula Pugh, Mary Richardson, Joy Solberg, Leslie Ward, and Anne Glenn White for lending us their ironing boards and coffee pots, their homes, hotel rooms, and spare bedrooms. Their generosity of spirit and their hospitality have helped us gather an ever-expanding community of fabulous women throughout the United States who are eager to redefine desire on their own terms.

We offer a huge round of applause to the 55 courageous and candid women who graciously agreed to be interviewed—you know who you are. Hurrahs to the more than 400 women who responded to our survey. By candidly answering our questionnaire and giving us your perspective, you made a major contribution to women's collective knowledge about sexuality and aging.

Hundreds of people—physicians, nurses, therapists, counselors, educators, and remarkable women—from all corners of the United States have attended our workshops and seminars and listened to our keynotes. Our work is stronger because of your interest and your ideas.

The Temple Beth Or Community in Everett, Washington, truly lit our way. Thank you, Sam Friedman, for inviting us to your bar mitzvah. We offer a special thanks to our ever-expanding mahjong group for relieving the tension and toasting our successes. We want to especially acknowledge Susan Cross, Melanie Field, Marilyn Glosser, Barb Ingram, Eileen Hinds, Ellie Hochman, Janet Karr, Rabbi Harley and Barbara Karz-Wagman, Kathie Roon, Vicki Romero, Nancy Sosnove, Vicky Schwartz, Sonia Siegel Vexler, Sandy Voit, Cheryl Waldbaum, and Janis Warner for scanning their Palm Pilots, their address books, and their memories to find women who would be receptive to participating in our research.

From one corner of the country to another, a cadre of creative folks—Grant Abbott, Jo Amundson, Donna Appel-Schramm, Dana Banks, Jo Ellen Bryant, Kanit Cottrell, Evie Dahm, Stephanie Davis, Ginny Greeno, Cathy Heffron, Rabbi Jay Heyman, Kaaren Johnson, Robin Jollay, Rhona Klein, Isabel Marker, Asunta Ng, Pam Peterson, Zora Pesio, Maggie Savage, Diana Sheridan, Elaine Tarone, Chris Volkmann, Jim and Carolyn Wartchow, and Penny Zimmerman—offered advice and enthusiastic contributions.

Special thanks goes to the early morning water aerobics classes at the Columbia Athletic Club at Juanita Bay, Kirkland, Washington, and the Mukilteo Washington YMCA, and to all women everywhere who dare to get up and get wet to get fit.

We have been fortunate to work with a talented group of associates who made our project a reality: Brett Malin and his staff at MR Data Corporation for the data input and the innumerable cross tabs; Nancy Hardwick and her staff at Hardwick Research, Mercer Island, Washington, for data analysis; Kathleen Florio for her editing skills and confidence in our abilities; Judy Reeves and Shana Hinds for their clerical help; and Jeff Tolbert, webmaster wizard. A special note of thanks goes to Peggy Hearn of Wallace O'Farrell for working with us to develop and market WB-50, our brand of personal lubricant for women beyond 50. We would also like to extend our thanks to Professor Lorraine Dennerstein, director of the Office for Gender and Health, Department of Psychiatry, the University of Melbourne, Melbourne, Australia, for help in developing one of our survey questions, and to Dr. Patti Ganz, whose important research has expanded our knowledge about women and cancer.

The Whidbey Island Writers Association and the Pacific Northwest Writers Association have served legions of writers. Thank you for teaching us how to pitch our work and hone our craft.

The University of Washington Department of Health Services, School of Public Health, and the University of Washington Department of Clinical Psychology taught us the necessary foundational skills and motivated us to expand on them.

AASECT (the Association of Sex Educators, Counselors and Therapists) is a tremendously important group of sexuality professionals who give us a platform for discussion. They honor us with their support.

Acknowledgments from Leah:

For more than 30 years, Coleen Belisle, Sherry Beckett, Marcella Brady, and Hob Osterlund have offered me a home in their hearts.

Their confidence, tears, laughter, advice, and editing capabilities nourish my soul. I am awed by our long-term friendship.

Doctor your highness Mary Richardson's indubitable faith and camaraderie are gifts beyond compare. Thank you.

Thank you to dear friends Michele Campbell, Ginny Daily, Victoria Galanti, Sondra Kornblatt, Jennifer Lego, Susan Levy, Suzie Rose-Jeltsch, Joy Solberg, Linda Sharpe, Anna Satenstein, and Debby Seaman for your guidance. You have come into my life throughout the past twenty-five years just when I needed you the most.

Thank you to my colleagues and physician friends Don Solberg, Lon Hatfield, Pat Heffron, and Bruce Amundson for practicing medicine in a way that makes a real difference in the lives of women. Your love, kindness, and support sustain me more than you could ever know.

And finally, I wish to thank the extraordinary men (and one boy) in my immediate family: my husband Phil Sandifer buoys my spirits and revs my engine, my son Sean Kliger offers unconditional love and computer wizardry, son Phil Sandifer keeps me laughing, brother-in-law Terry Parcheta cures my GERD, son-in-law Jeff Conwell shares his late harvest Riesling, and grandson Adam Sandifer supports my baseball habit. I am blessed by your support and love.

Acknowledgments from Deborah:

I am blessed by the wonderful women friends who have graced my life and supported me the whole length of the way: Colene McKee, Harriet Cannon, Suzanne Poppema, Barb Melinkovich, and Elizabeth Robinson, I love you all. My steadfast reading group—Judy and Kirk, Nancy and Carl, John and Suzanne—let's keep reading together forever.

Thank you to Robinson/Nedelman Psychological Associates, my professional home, and to all those women and men who have had the courage to examine the most vulnerable aspects of their lives with openness and optimism and who have been willing to trust me to act as their guide in the process.

I am especially grateful to Robin Gaudette and the women who work out at Synergy Personal Fitness, including Helen Kendall and Kay Peterson, who helped me get out of bed every morning, kept track of my progress in so many ways, and contributed their unique perspectives to this work.

My lifelong gratitude goes to Bryn Mawr College and her generous alumnae who taught me that being a woman has no limits.

My daughter, Eden—thank you for inspiring, challenging, and cheering me, always. A very special thank you goes to my cousin, Cheryl Sindell, with whom I am relearning the meaning of family. And thanks to Jane Criner, who is part of that family and a role model in her own right.

A number of others gave support in many varied ways: Kathy Fox, who gave me just the right place to write; Elizabeth Austen and Ellen Bass, poets whose work captures the experience of being a woman; and Heidi Rendall, who has always encouraged her patients to be knowledgeable participants in their health-care decisions.

My final, deepest thanks go to the amazing men in my life, all of whom believed in the value of this book from the very beginning. My father, Archie Nedelman (of blessed memory), who never wavered in his love and kept me laughing till the end; my husband, Mel Trenor, who is my anchor and my sail; and my son, Aaron Casson Nedelman Trenor, who expands my world on a daily basis. My love and gratitude are beyond measure.

Please forgive us if we've forgotten you—we are, after all, beyond 50—we couldn't have done this without you.

Introduction

It was a risky decision. Of course, any decision to marry involves a large risk, but planning an outdoor wedding in the Pacific Northwest in April is truly tempting fate. Happily, the day of the ceremony was one of those crystal-blue, cloudless jewels that Seattleites like to keep secret from Californians. Jane, the mother of the bride, was a close friend of both of ours. As we were ushered to our seats, we greeted several of our women friends who had also come to support Jane. We'd spent many hours over the last year listening to her describe the trials and tribulations of the various wedding decisions. We'd talked about her hopes for her daughter's future.

As the charming young bride joined her husband-to-be at the altar, the sexual energy between them was palpable. They were both attractive, energetic, and swooningly in love—no doubt about it. As the wedding march faded, we settled back into the white folding chairs. Leah leaned over and whispered, "How long do you think that passion is going to last?" Deborah shrugged her shoulders and sighed, grateful for a light breeze that eased her hot flash.

Following the ceremony, we joined our friends, all women of a certain age or older, at the wedding reception. We couldn't help wondering what they were thinking in the presence of all this youthful sexuality. Deborah approached Jane, and in a quiet moment asked, "So, how much have you told your daughter about how sexual desire changes as you age?" Jane emphatically said, "Nothing. Why burst her bubble? Anyway, what do I know?" Meanwhile, Leah dared to mention the topic of our curiosity to a circle of friends. "Deborah and I are thinking about writing a book on women's sexual desire after 50. What do you think?" The looks of shock and disbelief on their faces flabbergasted her. One dear friend, a gorgeous redhead who oozed sexuality, recoiled, "Oh, look, there's Jeri. I haven't seen her in ages," and scurried off. Another, an avant-garde artist, had a sudden and uncontrollable need to get to the bar for a refill. A third, a local politician, looked wonderingly at Leah and whispered, "Let me know the minute the book is out. And hurry up about it!" and then turned and hurried off to find her physician husband.

We ate our cake, dutifully scraping off the icing to maintain our figures. We offered our best wishes and made our way to the parking lot. "Gee, we sure touched a nerve, didn't we?" observed Deborah. Leah said, "They sure didn't want to pursue that conversation."

The contrast between what the newlyweds were experiencing and what the women over 50 at the reception seemed to be feeling was too dramatic to ignore. But what exactly was going on with our friends? Did they have the same negative attitudes and expectations about sexuality in older women that our culture has been promoting for decades? If they did, they weren't about to tell us in such a public setting. Fifteen years ago, nobody talked about menopause, either; now it's a musical. But sexual desire in aging women has remained a taboo subject in polite society. As long as grandmothers, mothers, nanas, bubbies, and aunties aren't openly talking about sexual desire, we will all remain in the dark. We decided it was time to turn on the light.

As health-care professionals for decades, we had more than a passing interest in the topic. Leah's career as a health educator, hospital executive, and advocate for women included teaching young women about sexuality, and Deborah had been a clinical psychologist and sex therapist treating women and couples for more than thirty years. Yet we still found ourselves facing our own sexual aging with doubt and confusion. Upon reaching menopause, we'd both begun to experience changes in our desire and our sexual self-esteem, and we wondered what our future would hold. We read a score of books and scads of magazine articles about menopause. But most of these talked about midlife zest and vaginal dryness and night sweats, or offered tips to make the sex act itself exciting. Often, they were written by medical doctors whose views were focused on dysfunction and pathology. We'd had several chats with our husbands. While supportive, they had their own questions. We ventured to ask a few really close friends what their experience had been like. But these conversations were short-lived and not very edifying. What we wanted was a resource to which women of a certain age could turn for an honest, revealing perspective on sexuality and aging. We wanted to know the unspoken truths. And we knew intuitively that other women wanted the same thing.

Had even one of our friends been willing to talk about herself that day at the wedding, we now know that her story would have given us only a small piece of the whole picture. The range of women's thoughts, feelings, and attitudes is vast. Everything from grief to relief to elation is part of the spectrum of women's reactions to changes in sexual desire. When we began our search for the unspoken truths in earnest, we didn't appreciate how broad that range is—we only knew that we had to turn to women themselves for the answers. We were determined to get a conversation going that would inform older women about what we were all going through sexually and what we could look forward to in the decades to come.

And were women across the country willing to talk to us? You bet. Over the next several years, hundreds of women from 50 to 95 talked to us about their own fruitless efforts to discover the unspoken truths about what to expect as they got older. Some whispered to us over the phone, fearful of their husbands overhearing, as we interviewed them; others huddled in small condos overlooking congested streets, wanting to know where their sexual desire fit into that vague continuum called the normal range. As we celebrated at the bar mitzvah of a friend's son, we again tried to get the conversation going. Once women heard about our project, we were deluged with questions: "Do other women know any more than I do about what to expect?" "Do other women tell you that they're surprised by what's happening to them?" "Do other women think they are weird?"

Because we did not want to focus on women who had identified themselves as sexually "dysfunctional," we decided against taking the traditional research route of using a pool of patients who visit physician offices or who seek out psychotherapy. Believing that we could expect a pretty low response rate if we mailed out questionnaires about sexuality to randomly selected older women, we tried a different approach. We developed an informal network of women across the country who assisted us in gathering information. Certainly our research was not a double-blind placebo-controlled study. We cannot claim that those who participated in our study are a random sample of the total population of women beyond 50, but we did reach women in 48 states and the District of Columbia. We made great attempts to assure more than a modicum of racial diversity. While we believe we reached a fairly decent cross section of Caucasian women, African-American women, Hispanic women, and Latinas, we were, and continue to be, dismayed that we were thwarted in our attempts to reach older Asian women, women from the Indian subcontinent, and Native American women. On average, the income and educational levels of the women we reached were somewhat higher than the norm. The majority of the women were mainstream Protestants and Catholics; a fair number were Jewish, and other theologies were also represented: one woman was a pagan, several were born-again Christians, a few labeled themselves as "recovering from organized religion" yet were profoundly spiritual. Unfortunately, not even one woman identified herself as a Muslim.

To collect our data, we utilized a three-pronged approach: a thirty-two question survey, in-depth interviews, and group discussions. During the first phase, we surveyed 408 women, including wives, mothers, grandmothers, childless widows, divorcees, women who had never married, lesbians, and bisexuals. We conducted telephone interviews with fifty-five women who volunteered to talk with us in greater depth about the effects of aging on their sexual desire and self-esteem. While most took place on the phone, we conducted a few face-to-face interviews, and a couple of women asked to write their own stories. One woman had been married for sixty-two years to her only sexual partner; another woman, recently married for the first time at age 57, had had more than 100 partners. The third approach we used was "What Color Is Your Sexual Desire?" house gatherings. These were informal discussion groups held in women's homes across the country. The hostess would invite 10 to 15 of her friends in our target age group to attend, and one or both of us would lead a discussion about the topic. We met with well over 100 women in homes across the country.

Since concluding the formal part of our study, we have continued to analyze our data, talk with older women through our workshops and seminars, and receive feedback from a survey posted on our website. While the stories and anecdotes from the women who participated are provocative, the statistics reinforce the unspoken truths and provide the hard data many in the health-care community—counselors, therapists, physicians, and sex educators—are looking for as they try to understand and treat older women. What we have learned from the perceptions and comments of remarkably candid women between the ages of 50 and 95 adds a wealth of information to the relatively scanty body of knowledge about older women's sexuality and self-esteem.

We continue to be astounded by the range of attitudes and emotions triggered by our research—our own, as well as those of other older women, and men, too. Women describe how the process of discussing their sexual desire and self-esteem has affected them. Repeatedly, we hear statements like Judith's: "I have never talked with anyone about my sexual desire since I went through menopause. I just thought there was nothing to say, but boy I was so wrong!" Some women talk about embracing a new sense of femininity and sexuality as they aged. And then there are the messages we receive via our website: "Let the world see that an older woman can be beautiful as she is, without artifice, without paint, without disguise. There is no need to make your lips red, nor your eyes black to be beautiful; the opposite is true." Women let us know that the options for aging sexually are infinite.

> We're nice Southern girls and we never discussed sex…the only problem is we're over 60 now, isn't it about time?
>
> —*Marsha, a single librarian, Elyria, Ohio*

You—or the people who love you—may have noticed some vague shift in your desire. Perhaps you are afraid that this is the start of an unrelenting downward slide and find your sexual self-esteem plummeting. Or maybe the level of your desire has been higher since you turned 50. You might be a bit concerned that this is a sign that you're going to be one of those old women who are ridiculed for being sexually interested when you're supposed to be sidelined to a rocking chair. Or perhaps, the expectations you have for the next 20 or 30 years are that you'll dry up sexually and that will be the end of intimacy. Without a road map that tells all of us what is coming next, we fall back on the myths our society perpetuates. We encourage you to reject the limitations that corral older women's sexuality and sing your own song—even if you sing a bit off key like we do! This book is designed to help you chart your course for sexual aging and to reclaim your sexual self-esteem. We want it to be your ticket to a grand, later-life adventure.

Warmly,

Leah Kliger and Deborah Nedelman
September 2005

Truth #1

Older Women Can't Be Pigeonholed

How to Assess Your Own Sexual Truth Beyond 50

Amid the clamor and clutter of everyday life, Susan's pesky inner voice had been easy to ignore. But the other night when Richard, whom she adored, was in an amorous mood and she once again felt totally unresponsive, she could no longer brush aside her fears. Several years ago, with the hot flashes and night sweats and all the other discomforts of menopause, she wasn't surprised—or, to be honest, distressed—that she didn't feel much sexual desire. But what did trouble her, even back then, was the awareness that she had somehow crossed an invisible barrier and had entered the "matronly" zone. Her body had just sort of slumped—gone south, as they say. It's not that she had ever thought that her body was perfect, but she had at least felt sexually appealing most of her adult life.

Susan had enjoyed sex with Richard for the last 25 years, and with a few other guys before him. She hadn't thought of herself as an exceptionally sexual person, though. There were so many other parts of her life that she'd always valued—her career, for one. Being a librarian at the university was a stimulating and fulfilling job; sure, it had its ups and downs, and some days the bureaucracy really got to her, but on the whole she loved her work and her colleagues. Music had always given her a great deal of pleasure, and she still treasured her time at the piano. The kids were on their own now, and she felt good about her relationships with them. She and Richard were great companions, always had been. It was just that that bond they used to reinforce with sex wasn't as resilient somehow. It seemed she'd lost something—something that felt like a part of her identity.

She thought about the other women she knew who were in their 60s or even older and wondered if they had felt this way in their 50s. Her mother, of course, had never told her a single helpful thing about sex. It just wasn't a subject she'd been able to broach when Susan was younger, and now, in her 80s, that was not likely to change. "Anyway, what's the point?" Susan thought. "Mom surely stopped feeling like a sexual person long ago. So is this the beginning of the end of that feeling for me, too?"

Cultural Myths

Popular notions about older women's sexual identity seldom extend beyond dry vaginas and power surges. Sure, people toss around jokes about mental lapses. Books about menopause turn up on bestseller lists. Illustrated manuals extol the virtues of acrobatic sex acts, using models with gray hair to appeal to older couples. But questions about how a woman beyond 50 can feel good about her sexuality— wherever she may be in the broad spectrum of desire—are met with deafening silence.

We know it's damn hard to hang onto sexual self-confidence when, as mature women, we are marginalized as asexual, unattractive, and undesirable. How many of us have not felt a flicker of resentment when chirpy young waiters patronize us by referring to us as "ma'am"? Who among us doesn't cringe when we see how older women are portrayed in commercials? Even in the doctor's office, we're dumped into the "dysfunctional" category when we grumble that our sexual desire has evaporated. Mature women who are treated as if they are invisible find it hard to feel sexy!

The 44 million women over age 50 who live in the United States today have heaps of womanly wisdom and confidence when it comes to child rearing, career building, money, and even the sex act itself. But few roadmaps guide women at midlife and beyond when it comes to sexual self-esteem. Women of a certain age face a waxing and waning of desire, changing relationships, debilitating societal myths, and their own conflicting emotions. They question whether they are sexually typical or some kind of aberration.

Experiences of sexual desire and aging are individual and unpredictable. Although many older women are less interested in sex, some discover a sexual self-assurance that is more rewarding than what they experienced in their youth. And these women aren't necessarily partnered. They use their creativity (and sometimes their sex toys) to help revitalize their allure, achieve self-sufficiency, and power up during the last five decades of life.

Negotiating new sexual terrain can be intimidating. At this stage of life, one size—a new pill, a new diet, or a new relationship—doesn't fit all. The nature of the interaction between sexual desire and self-worth is complicated. Many of us have some combination of stiff joints, minds like sieves,

> Sexual self-esteem comes because of your belief that you're worth being treated with respect. Sexual liaisons are tests of your resolve to be treated well. It's hard to maintain this resolve when your body wants to "play" while your mind and your gut tell you to walk away.
>
> —*Anita, 61, songwriter, Kansas*

and leaking bladders. Wrinkles, chin hairs, the pull of gravity, and myriad psycho-social factors can leave even the most "together" woman in tears. Women who gleefully welcomed the freedom from earlier sexual demands may run smack dab into Viagra-induced erect husbands whose disappointment at being rebuffed is too blatant to ignore. Or these same men may have an adverse reaction to the drugs and dismiss any further intimacy with their wives. Women who have little sexual desire wonder if they can be healthy and maintain positive sexual self-esteem without ever having sex.

> My mother told me to lay there like a lox.
>
> —*Rose, 78, Brooklyn, New York*

Is it any surprise that *discouraged* and *lost* are words that come to mind when older women think about maintaining or reclaiming sexual self-confidence? Incessant media messages reinforce the myth that sexuality is only for the young and that a woman's fiftieth or certainly sixtieth birthday signals the end of magnetism. TV commercials feature older women touting pharmaceutical remedies for constipation or dental adhesive, or portray them as sexless grandmothers whose life revolves around taking the grandkids to the park. Magazine covers bombard readers with the benefits of looking young—promoting plastic surgery and Botox® as ways to get and keep a man, suggesting that unless women look like Hollywood's image of beauty they're not worth looking at...let alone relating to.

Commonly, if a woman in her 60s or 70s or 80s is sexually interested, she is often categorized as pathetic and inappropriate. Tune in to a cable channel offering reruns and catch an episode of the 1980s sitcom *The Golden Girls*. The stars, Beatrice Arthur, Betty White, Rue McClanahan, and Estelle Getty, are energetic, fun, and have a zest for life. Yet the show continually reinforces old stereotypes. McClanahan's Blanche, the youngest and "prettiest," is depicted as one-dimensional: overly partial to men and wild sex. More often than not, the punch lines revolve around her sexuality, depicting it as ridiculous. As baby boomers turn 50 and 60, these "over-the-hill" images may change, but we have a long way to go.

Defining Desire

What is normal sexuality in the older woman? For that matter, what is sexual desire once a woman is beyond 50? "I don't know how to define sexual desire, but I know it when I feel it," said Liz, a perfectly coiffed, regal, and articulate 56-year-old book editor. We met Liz in Florida at the first in a series of "What Color Is Your Sexual Desire?" discussion groups we held. Her statement left us stymied. At her age and given her profession, if she couldn't define it, who could? Dictionary definitions of sexual desire focus on the sex act and childbearing. But women beyond 50 are past their reproductive years, and some may not have had sex in years. Scientific literature and self-help books offer little more than confusing and contradictory descriptions of postmenopausal sexual desire and barely mention the notion of sexual self-esteem. Most advise women that regaining their lost desire is paramount to leading a healthy life. Doctors are often too busy, have too little training, or are too embarrassed to discuss the topic with a partially clad woman sitting on the exam table who reminds them of their own mother.

As women of a certain age ourselves, we know that the sexual desire and self-esteem we felt in our 20s and 30s is not what most of us are experiencing today. If we continue to focus on youth-oriented perspectives, we miss out on who we are now. It's a bit like trying to stuff a 59-year-old foot into a pointy-toed shoe worn to the high school prom—it might fit initially, but wear it very long and it's sure to cause pain. It makes a lot more sense to find a new style. It's time to develop our own style and definition of sexuality based on the

honest experiences of women—not on the stunted role models society promotes.

As we began our search for the real picture of older women's sexuality, we recognized that the term *sexual desire,* although part of our
common vocabulary, has a differ-
ent meaning for each woman.
In fact, we asked hundreds of
women beyond 50, from all walks
of life, "How would you personally define *sexual desire?*" Not
surprisingly, we got a wide range
of responses.

> Sexual desire is some distinct
> energy that permeates through-
> out my body in ebbs and flows—
> unhindered by time or place, it
> seems to have a force of its own.
>
> —*Anitra, 56, physical therapist,*
> *Atlanta, Georgia*

The most common definition
of *desire* we heard is similar to that
given by Brenda, a 65-year-old bisexual who lives in Chicago: "A
woman's desire tends to be stimulated less by visual stimulus in a vacuum, that is, by seeing a good-looking but anonymous body, than by
elements of attentiveness, consideration, emotional generosity, 'courtly
romance.' It's really the desire to be close to someone."

Even subtle differences in meaning are important in understanding women's attitudes and perceptions. Older women typically
talked about desire and self-worth as a complex experience. Joan, a
58-year-old school principal from Missoula, Montana, says, "My
desire may be less intense, but also slower and more prolonged. I do
not define sexual desire as simply wanting to have sex. It's like a
magnificent stew of my entire being." One American woman of
Japanese ancestry told us, "Feeling desire and acting on it is like a
meeting with God."

As we accumulated the personal definitions of *sexual desire* from
older women, we found, in addition to many differences, a number
of commonalities. Our further research reinforced the power of
these themes.

The Five Qualities of Desire

1. Desire Is Mysterious: What's coming next?

Generally, the first question we're asked at our seminars and workshops is "What can I expect to happen to my sexuality in the future?" Our study revealed that women simply do not know what might happen to their sexuality as they age. In spite of their experience up to this point, women are all over the map about what's coming next. Although 56 percent have already experienced a drop in desire, only 39 percent expect a further decrease, 33 percent expect no change, 13 percent expect an increase, and 15 percent don't know what to expect.

Expectations can be self-fulfilling prophecies. If a woman expects that her level of sexual desire will be high as she ages, such an prediction can set her up to focus on her sexuality and even to act on her feelings. In fact, it may make a woman feel healthier and happier to be sexually active, thus enhancing her sexual assurance. (See Chapter 4.) But if she expects that her desire will drop over time, her sexual self-esteem will likely be negatively affected. Buying into a belief that a woman can't lead a satisfying life without much desire today is a setup for a dreary tomorrow.

2. Desire Is Diverse: "Normal" covers a wide range

Our findings confirmed what numerous other studies have shown: for many women, desire tends to diminish with age. Fifty-six percent of the women we surveyed said, "My sexual desire is less than it used to be." At the same time, 40 percent said their desire was either the same as ever or was greater now than it used to be. Four percent of women told us they simply didn't know about their current level of sexual desire. This last statistic may well be a result of the fact that this topic is so hidden—many women told us that they had never been asked about their sexual desire before.

Physicians are just as perplexed. They are rushed and generally lack training in sexuality. They often take a singularly unhelpful approach toward mature women who turn to them for guidance. For example, at her annual exam a woman may say, "I just don't give a damn about sex anymore." The doctor's response is apt to be something like, "You should, because it is important for your life quality." And if she says, "Well, is it okay to stop making love if you don't feel like it?" her doctor may say, "No, you shouldn't stop—regardless of apathy."

This notion that there is a single best way for older women to handle their sexuality runs totally counter to what we have learned. Scores of women we talked to described having very full, exciting, creative lives without having any sexual desire—or sexual activity, for that matter. Sometimes they told us, "I'm just not aroused. It seems like such work!" Some, like Hannah, attributed this drop in desire to a lack of hormones: "What still boggles my mind, even after these last eight years or so of no hormones, is that sex doesn't even enter into my mind. I might even have the desire if the thought would occur, but it doesn't. I work out, and my body looks pretty good. I still have the knowledge and confidence; I just don't have the desire. I don't get horny anymore."

For some women, desire seems to be a steady state. Margie, a 55-year-old nurse from Florida, wrote us, "I've been with my partner now for 16 years, and the highs and lows of my desire have leveled off. My desire is always pretty much the same."

On the other hand, Lulu, a divorced saleswoman in her 70s from Antioch, Ohio, wrote us, "My desire has increased, but I have no partner! Could it be that absence makes the heart grow fonder?"

To learn more about the women who find that they would rather be "picking apples" than engaging in sexual activities, turn to

Chapter 3. For insight into women whose desire has surged, turn to Chapter 4.

3. Desire Is Unpredictable: It ebbs and flows

A consistent theme emerged when older women characterized their sexual desire: desire waxes and wanes over time. Women talked about periods when their desire was particularly low. Sometimes they could identify a stressor that seemed to explain this, but other times it would drop for no apparent reason. Occasionally, they would experience heightened desire. Many times this occurred at the beginning of a new relationship; other times it just happened. Women in long-term marriages talked about this variability, as did women who had been single for most of their lives. Widows experienced it, and so did lesbians in committed relationships.

With her honey-blond, shoulder-length hair beginning to show a little gray, Andrea, an energetic 54-year-old preschool teacher, has many qualities that endear her to the parents of her young charges. With a little encouragement, she mentioned that her natural exuberance and zest for life has attracted six sexual partners since she was 18. Married for fifteen years and now divorced, her life is full of evenings out with her many friends. Andrea is involved in her church and loves attending art shows. The ups and downs of her sexual desire have been apparent to her throughout her adult life. Sometimes she has actively pursued efforts to increase her desire, but at other times she's been comfortable just letting it be: "Well, I am sort of in the doldrums right now. I am sort of okay with it, but I don't want to see it just dwindle off and slide into nothing, either. However, I am not really sure what to do about it—perhaps pursuing this friendship that I am beginning with this man, or maybe with someone else will make a difference. I don't want my sexual desire to go away, and yet I don't feel motivated to cultivate it right now."

> Desire has multiple meanings: how sexual I feel about my own self, do I feel like I am attractive sexually, do I feel some urge, how I feel about sex.
>
> —*Lisa, 58, self-described "confused Lutheran" from Iowa*

Tisha, a vibrant, well-educated Latina professional in her late 50s, lives in a charming row house in South San Francisco. She has been divorced for four years from a husband who tore down her self-esteem throughout their twenty-year marriage. It's taken Tisha several years to get beyond the anger and grief that overwhelmed her during the lengthy and bitter divorce proceedings. Now in a new and much more passionate relationship, Tisha reflected on how her desire had shifted over time. "Especially after the divorce, I felt I really didn't have much self-esteem. I wasn't feeling like I had any desire, any libido, or that I was desirable to anybody else. But that feeling has come back. I know it goes up and down. When it's down I don't feel quite content, if I were to put a finger on it. And it has nothing to do with the sexual act. It is part of my being. It is like there is something missing from me."

4. Desire Is Responsive: Women measure desire in the context of a relationship

For a large number of the mature women with whom we spoke, sexual desire was something they recognized only in relation to a sexual partner. Many were reluctant to admit it, but they acknowledged that the primary factor that arouses their own desire is feeling that they are attractive to another person. Numerous women told us that their desire mirrors their partner's, that if he (or she) isn't interested in them, they didn't feel sexual. Diane, who is in her early 50s, told us, "It's the rush of a sexy man that I respond to. If there's no guys around my desire fades away."

Many widows told us that when their husbands died, their desire evaporated. Teresa, a 78-year-old Protestant widow of Irish extraction, speaks for countless widows: "Well, I am reconciled to the fact that I don't have a mate. I am not looking for a mate. I am quite happy and content. My husband and I had a great sexual life together, and as far as I know he never strayed, and I know for a fact that I never strayed. It was his attention that turned me on. Now that he's gone, I'm busy doing other things and don't think much about desire. About once a month though, I have a dream about being on an island somewhere and my husband is there and I'm aroused sexually. But, most of the time, my thoughts are elsewhere."

Ingrid, a 55-year-old who has never married, describes this responsive quality of desire: "What makes me feel excited is to know that I am exciting to a man. So I guess my own attractiveness becomes my own turn-on, ultimately. It comes back to me feeling attractive to a man."

Many of the women we heard from told us they had begun to reevaluate what makes them sexually attractive to their partners. It's a given that another person's attention is a powerful validator. It's an ego boost. But if a woman's sexual self-worth is totally tied to the feeling that others find her attractive, it's a no-win proposition. She'll end up feeling disgruntled and even depressed, rather than positive about the future. Women talked to us about longing to be free of the "sexy woman" stereotype imposed on them for as long as they could remember. They knew that despite crinkles or saggy knees, their sexual responsiveness is really a matter of the heart, not of the eye.

5. Desire Is Invigorating: Sexual desire can increase, even after 80

We discovered that not only do individual women experience ebbs and flows in their desire and sexual confidence over time, but also that women in general are likely to see notable shifts of desire throughout the last five decades of life. In fact, 19 percent of women in our study who were over 80 said that their desire was greater than it used to be. This was a higher percentage than women in their 50s or 60s or 70s.

Those who volunteered for our study represent only a portion of this older age group. Perhaps they are the risk-takers; they may be somewhat healthier than many who have celebrated their 80th birthdays. Health certainly matters when it comes to sexual desire, but it is important to know that women over 80 who are relatively healthy can be very passionate, even if their desire had been less noticeable at other points in their life.

Our chances of living into our 80s and even our 90s are greater than ever. We will have choices that our mothers and our grandmothers never dreamed of. Although sexual desire and sexual activity are not essential components of sexual self-esteem, our image of old age can change if we embrace the possibility of passionate sex at 85. We may not wish to be sexually involved with a partner once we are octogenarians, but it is important to know that women are capable of fervor and sensuality at that stage in life. Understanding that sexual self-esteem is a vital part of our later years is crucial to grasping our full potential as women.

> My husband's health had precluded any significant sexual activity for several years before his death. So when I met Roger, I was shocked by my response when a tentative kiss initiated by me sent an electric current through me from head to toe. Those reactions remain current (no pun intended)!
>
> —*Colette, 85, widowed at 70*

Mildred's story illustrates what it means to be sexually revitalized. A hardy, somewhat reticent New Englander, she's been widowed for seven years. Spurred by her need to talk about the changes she's experienced, she called us back a number of times to clarify her story and to offer us encouragement and support. She spoke of how she had bought into some of the myths about older women's desire and how discouraging that had been to her self-confidence. Her marriage to her husband of forty-six years had not been fulfilling to her sexually. She had always believed that her own desire was very low, especially after her doctor labeled her as "frigid." After her husband's death, Mildred began exploring creative outlets that she had denied herself earlier. A music lover, she began listening to a wide variety of styles and going to concerts her husband would not have appreciated. In this process she discovered a love for jazz—and for a jazz musician.

Herbert was drawn to her vitality and adventurous personality. Together they found that Mildred was far from frigid. "Now I am fine. I really feel comfortable. My lover is in Paris for a month right now, but we talk on the phone every now and then. When he gets back, you know, we will be right back there with our relationship, and the time apart doesn't seem to make a difference. I would have been going overboard if that had been true in my marriage, but that was just the anxiety of not feeling easy with my own self, whatever my sexual level was. Back then, whenever my desire was not high, it meant something. I have found out that was wrong; it was like a hypochondriac's attitude. These days it doesn't take all that much to arouse me." Does it surprise you to learn that Mildred is 83 years old?

Women told us a great deal about sexual desire and their self-worth. We learned how multifaceted and complex it is. How women feel about themselves is so fundamental to their well-being that it can even affect brain size, as recent research has shown. Dr. Sonia Lupien of McGill University in Montreal studied the brain scans of ninety-two senior citizens over a period of fifteen years. She discovered that the brains of those who had low self-worth were up to a fifth smaller in size them those who had more positive attitudes!

We also recognized that a woman's level of desire does not

necessarily correlate with how she feels about herself as a sexual be-ing. There is clearly something more intrinsic to how a woman sees herself that determines her ability to feel assured and confident as she ages. We began looking closely at the concept of sexual self-esteem.

"I'm having difficulty defining sexual self-esteem," said Evie. "If it means do I think I'm attractive, at age 92 I know men won't make passes. But I don't care. I feel good about myself. In my 50s my sex-ual self-esteem dropped to zero when I walked past a construction site and not one man whistled. Now I don't expect whistles. I'd rate my self-esteem a ten, but am not real sure how'd I rate my sexual self-esteem. After Fred, my late husband, died, a handsome, sexy, divorced man in his late 50s who Fred and I had known for twenty-some years, told me he loved me and asked me to marry him.

"I, at age 89 and old enough to be his grandma, was pleased and flattered and tempted to say yes; then reason took over. Why would a handsome young man with a high-paying job want to marry an old woman like me? It couldn't be for my brains, my wit, or my voluptuous bod. No, it must be because I own a home valued at half a million. So I said no. We are still friends and on e-mail together."

In spite of her white hair and stooped shoulders, Evie remains a sparkling presence—a person who draws others to her. It isn't hard to recognize in her the giggling flapper who helped her young husband ferry discarded biplanes from Europe to Palestine at the end of WWII. Long widowed, today she lives alone in a bungalow near the beach and spends much of her day at the computer, connecting with her wide circle of friends. Now in her ninth decade, Evie is undoubtedly a sexual being with vitality and warmth. Her life and attitude certainly do not fit the pattern our culture typically assigns to aging women.

Is Evie an anomaly? If she is, does it mean the rest of us are des-tined to ride a roller coaster that sends our self-confidence through dizzying ups and downs in the last five decades of our lives? Is there a path that will allow us to maintain a secure level of sexual self-esteem in spite of the disorientation that comes with the all-encompassing transformation of post-menopausal aging?

By listening to the life stories of older women, we accumulated lots of evidence that those who have weathered the storms of menopause and the succeeding decades and survived with positive self-esteem possess some important attributes. We have begun to think of these attributes as the essential ingredients in the recipe for sexual self-confidence beyond 50. They each add a necessary flavor, though the proper blending will vary for every woman.

The Four Ingredients of Sexual Self-Esteem

1. A jumbo portion of comfort with your body

One of the questions we're frequently asked: "Since I've gotten older, I'm embarrassed if my husband sees me naked; am I alone in this?" Reevaluating common definitions of sexual attractiveness and finding freedom from the sexy woman labels imposed by a youth-oriented culture is not just wishful thinking. You can rid yourself of the perceptions that trap you, but it takes work. You'll reap enormous rewards if you disengage from the competitive game of self-evaluation and learn to honestly cherish who you are today. You may want to have a little nip or tuck taken, or you may choose to go au naturale. Perhaps you spend hours at the gym or find the sensuality of a massage gives you reason to value your body. Regardless of your approach, we recommend that you reexamine your internal definition of attractiveness. Do your best to ignore the societal pressure we all feel to gauge our personal value by artificial standards of physical beauty.

Annette has made peace with her body at age 60. Being sexy by society's standards was very important to her when she was younger. She used to struggle with weight issues and would constantly compare her body to those of younger women. After fighting the battle with gravity and confronting a more threatening enemy—cancer—Annette took stock of her life. Today she has a more forgiving and accepting attitude toward herself. "My sexuality is transforming into a sensual intimacy. I am expecting to continue to enjoy whatever, however my body is. To enjoy it as it is. And because I know we do get illnesses, I just want to appreciate my body as it is."

2. A taste for the beauty in life

Numerous women repeated this theme: as their sexuality went through modifications, their creativity blossomed. "I've swapped sex for creativity, said Shelly, who, at 59, has been married to Ed for almost thirty-five years. "I opened a fabric shop about seven years ago. For the first several years, I spent the better part of every day just selling fabric. Then I realized what I most enjoyed was talking to the women who were quilters. So I branched out—began ordering more quilting supplies, then I started teaching classes. Now women are flocking to the shop, and I can't wait to get out of bed in the morning. My husband and I still share a bit of sexual intimacy but not nearly the same level of acrobatics as before. We've found a comfortable position, and we keep that position all the time."

Other women described their increased appreciation for the sensual in everyday life and how important it has become to surround themselves with beauty. For many, their 50s, 60s, and 70s were the decades when they finally gave themselves permission to explore creative impulses and try new outlets, from glassblowing to playing the drums. They found that taking the time to indulge in whatever form of expression is appealing can lead to newfound sources of pleasure and satisfaction. We heard this from Diana, a 63-year-old hospital administrator in Iowa: "I now find myself being much more appreciative of nature, of music, of colors, of beauty in general than I ever did before. I find intimacy in nature, in quiet spaces, and in my garden. It's no longer the big excitement of my youth, but the serenity satisfies my soul."

3. Ample servings of each of the following: autonomy, assertiveness, and authenticity

Once women celebrate their 50th birthdays, having a sexual partner for life is no longer the focus for self-definition that it once was. Rather than getting bogged down in societal expectations and roles, what becomes important for many women is the ability to value and respect the life choices they've made and to take responsibility for creating their own reality. For example, after her divorce, Julie is living alone for the first time in her life...and she is very aware of her own sexual desire: "I have always had a healthy sexual appetite. Currently I am divorced and am not dating. Would I welcome a chance to have a relationship? You bet! The difference is I'm a lot pickier at 53 than I was at 23!"

• **Autonomy.** Freeing yourself to make choices in your own best interests is the heart of self-sufficiency. Taking control over your own life doesn't necessarily mean living it alone. Many women who were in long-term marriages or had life partners expressed the importance of seeing their lives as their own without allowing their partner's needs to be the primary motivation for their decisions.

Jan, a Baptist from Alabama, puts this concept in perspective: "At this stage in life I am less concerned with sex in a relationship than with companionship and compatibility. Sexual desire was not the primary reason I married 38 years ago; nor was it a factor in my divorce 23 years ago. And it may not be the most important reason for involvement in future relationships. I am my own best friend."

• **Assertiveness.** Acknowledging that your life experience is extraordinarily significant, and allowing yourself to flex your muscles and feel your power, is a crucial component of self-esteem. Numerous women told us they had learned to stand up for what they know to be true in spite of the pressure to retreat into matronly invisibility. It is not a given that once your waistline swells and the wrinkles appear your sexual self-worth vanishes.

Glenda, a lovely 58-year-old African-American woman who attended one of our discussion groups in Los Angeles, gave us her impressions of one of the other participants: "I was so struck by Candy. Although her husband is this powerful minister, she exudes her own strength. She seems to have found a way to be herself rather than being just 'the wife,' and, boy, is she sexy! She's following her own path. How she operates gives much joy to others, but it doesn't diminish her personal power."

• **Authenticity.** The process of self-examination you began in your early years leads to the courage to be your own true self in your later years. Being brave enough to abandon your fears, admit your vulnerabilities, and quit hiding behind false pretenses is not easy. Authenticity is the most difficult ingredient to attain, yet it is so often what separates a truly confident, sexually secure older woman from one who feels disoriented in her aging body. For an authentic woman, personal honesty and self-acceptance beautify her more than cosmetics ever could.

4. A good dose of humor

Humor is the glue that preserves sexual sanity in the face of societal and personal pressures. The house gatherings and seminars we hold around the country echo with phenomenal good cheer (facilitated in part by big doses of chocolate). The attendees often tell us that they never expected to be talking aloud about their sexual desire at this point in their lives, but the infectious laughter makes it not only possible, but a downright joy.

For example, on a balmy January day in Clearwater, Florida, we asked the group "What color is your sexual desire?" Sharon answered, "Blue." And Dana, seated next to her, said, "Yeah, right—once in a blue moon!" At another winter gathering, this one in chilly Spokane, Washington, Madeline knew that the "hue" that turned her on was Hugh Grant. And, as Beatrice said when we asked her how she dealt with the changes in her sexual desire that aging had brought: "First I laugh about it and then my husband laughs along with me. It's certainly better than the alternative!"

The Green Grocer

Three old ladies were sitting side by side in their nursing home, reminiscing. The first lady recalled shopping at the green grocer's and demonstrated with her hands the length and thickness of a cucumber she could buy for a penny.

The second old lady nodded, adding that onions used to be much bigger and cheaper also, and demonstrated the size of two big onions she could buy for a penny apiece.

The third old lady remarked, "I can't hear a word you're saying, but I remember the guy you're talking about."

Assessing Your Own Truth

It's not surprising that aging brings changes in sexual desire and self-esteem. But often we don't consider how those changes may benefit us. Commonly, we continue to judge our level of functioning by those youthful standards that popular culture endorses rather than appreciating the growth that comes with maturity. We may also compare ourselves to what our sisters or cousins or best friends are experiencing. This can lock us into self-defeating patterns that negatively affect sexual self-esteem. But each individual is unique. Your host of experiences is singular. By examining what is really happening to your sexual desire and self-esteem, you can begin to break out of this spiral of negative expectation.

If you are a woman of 50 or beyond, take a few minutes to consider the following questions. You may wish to write your answers down in a journal, or, if that's not your style, think about them while you're washing your hair or gardening or walking the dog.

We encourage you to keep your responses handy as you read this book. These questions are designed to boost your level of awareness and help you gain greater insight into both your past and

What's the Status of Your Sexual Self-Esteem?

1. What is your definition of sexual self-esteem?

2. On a scale of 1 to 10, with 1 being lousy and 10 being fantastic, how's your sexual self-esteem today?

3. Has this changed from what it was five years ago, or even one year ago? How do you feel about these changes? Are the changes you've noticed a problem for you?

4. What are some of the factors that have affected your sexual self-esteem as you've aged? Has your body image, your energy level, or your lifestyle changed?

5. Are any of these factors within your control? If so, what, if anything, do you want to do about them? What could you do to help your sexual self-esteem become more positive?

your future sexuality. They can also serve as great conversation-starters. (If you need a guide to begin these conversations, check out Chapter 8.)

These questions have no right or wrong answers, and you won't receive a grade. What's true for you is all that matters. As you review your responses, look for patterns. You may be feeling great about your sexual self-esteem and can identify some of the factors. Perhaps you are in a new relationship and are having the best sex of your life. If so, you may wish to bond with the women whose stories are described in Chapter 4. If, on the other hand, you find yourself acknowledging that your sexual self-esteem has plunged in the past few years, don't despair. Scores of women in this book share their approaches to coping with just such a drop in confidence. Finally, if your answers leave you asking "What's the next step?" turn to Chapter 9 and check out Leila's manifesto for a new sexual order for women beyond 50. After you've finished this book and had a conversation or two with your husband or partner, a friend, your mother, or your daughter, review your answers; they may have changed.

We urge you to keep an open mind and shed narrow labels. You'll find that you are not alone—millions of older women have struggled to understand their own sexual transformations. Every day 5,000 American women celebrate their 50th birthdays. We are a huge presence. Together we have the power to change how society views us as well as how we view ourselves.

Truth #2

Sexy Is Different After 50

How to Reclaim Your Body Image on Your Own Terms

Mary stood at the bathroom sink, transfixed by the image before her. Her mouth foamy with toothpaste, the sparkle of peppermint awakening her senses, she was jolted by her reflection. "What's happened to me?" She thought as she appraised the dark circles under her eyes and her sagging chin. As a young, self-confident woman, Mary had expected that by the time she reached 54 she would be deaf to the relentless drumbeat of commercials and media images that attempt to manipulate women's attitudes about their own beauty. She'd never worn much makeup and always thought that when the time came, she'd be perfectly happy with lines and wrinkles.

Mary had always felt blessed that her smooth skin stretched

> My idea of myself as an attractive person has really changed. I can be walking in the woods and just experiencing the rain falling and the wet smells. I become aware that my body is responding to that sensuality. It's like my body wakes up. It's not about how I look but how I feel.
>
> —*Kathy, 56, divorced, Minnesota*

over her high cheekbones. Her wiry figure meant that she had been "carded" well into her 30s. But things had begun to change. In the past year, she'd taken to wearing slimming black pantsuits. On the advice of her hairdresser, she'd had her long hair clipped short.

On one aborted shopping trip, Mary had scurried out of Nordstrom after being thoroughly disgusted by a glimpse of her cellulite while trying on bathing suits. Even though she'd been exercising for years, the word *dumpy* echoed in her brain when she caught her image reflected in a shop window. It had been years since her weekly trip to the grocery store required a stop along the feminine hygiene aisle. Obviously, she'd moved on to a new stage in life.

At one of our discussion groups Mary and several of her friends described their mixed reactions to the cessation of their menstrual cycles. Some viewed the end of their reproductive years as a significant loss, while others gleefully celebrated the termination of the monthly curse. But it was all the other physical changes that

Old Friends

Two elderly ladies had been friends for many decades. Over the years, they had shared all kinds of activities and adventures. Lately, their activities had been limited to meeting a few times a week to play cards.

One day, they were playing cards when one looked at the other and said, "Now don't get mad at me…I know we've been friends for a long time…but I just can't think of your name! I've thought and thought, but I can't remember it. Please tell me what your name is."

Her friend glared at her. For at least three minutes she just stared. Finally she said, "How soon do you need to know?"

had come along with "the change" that really gave them pause. They talked about feeling defeated by their creaky joints, loss of sexual desire, and expanding waistlines. They whined about lack of energy, sleeplessness, and night sweats. They even told of night-mares dominated by the silhouettes of frumpy, asexual, gray-haired matrons fighting for recognition.

Mary is certainly not alone in her battle with her changing body. When asked "Which factors have had a negative impact on your sexual desire since turning 50?" more than 51 percent of women in our study listed "changes in body image." Many other factors were also identified, but none of them was endorsed by such a high percentage of re-spondents. Long-held habits of self-deprecation, critical body analysis, and unfavorable media portrayals eat away at older women's sexual self-esteem and, for many, at the ability to feel sexual desire. Wendy, a 55-year-old Iowa farm worker told us, "I'm 5 feet 1¹/₂ inches and prob-ably 30 pounds overweight at this point, and that has affected how I feel sexually. I mean I don't get dressed in front of my husband! I don't want to do that, I feel like he's going to look at me...and I don't want anybody else seeing me."

> ...I would look at older women, and if they were attractive I would think of them as possibly having sexual relationships. And if they were plain and unattractive—a grandmother who bakes and has a big lap to sit in, with gray hair—I would think no, she probably isn't interested much in sex.
>
> —*Roberta, 52, Roanoke, Virginia*

As we age, we all begin to see that face that dwells deeper within us—the look of our older relatives. The shift can feel as if your body is betraying you by revealing the heredity you had always wished to deny. If we think of those who passed their genes to us as over-the-hill, sexless beings, seeing their DNA in our bodies can be quite humbling. Right along with the ability to curl your tongue, your beautiful voice, or your talent in mathematics come the physical patterns of wear that distinguish your body and identify you as one of your clan: there are those neck wrinkles just like your aunt's, the cellulite your mother carried but you had recoiled from, your grand-mother's jowls.

Perhaps you are a much more active woman than your mother was, or you take better care of yourself than your hardworking grandmothers ever had time to do. If part of the physical legacy you have been given includes a tendency toward heart disease or diabe-tes, for example, your efforts to care for your body can make a huge difference in your overall health. These choices can make you a healthier person, but they can't prevent your body from showing some changes with age. Or possibly your mother, your aunt, or your grandmother is a woman whose lifestyle choices you emulate, who has aged as you hope to do. In that case, you may be grateful for your hered-ity. But you may still be dis-tressed by more subtle signs of age—you find your body doesn't move as easily as it used to, you tire more quickly, or there is less sensation when you are touched in a sexual way.

> I have always had a very, very positive body image. I was always very happy with the way I looked. In the past year I am much more dissatisfied, I am carrying a few more pounds than I like and noticing that I am losing tone and, you know, because of gravity, I'm droopy—my face is droopy, my breasts are not as up as they used to be. So I am much more critical of the way I look naked. And before I just thought I had a terrific body....
>
> —*Jackie, 54, Coeur d'Alene, Idaho*

Our bodies go through an undeniable transformation. From the predominant perspective of our culture, that is, through the eyes of men, these changes typically disqualify us from the category of sexy, appealing women. And sadly, when we recognize these changes in ourselves, we all too often bow out of the running. Our culture certainly makes a clear distinction between young, fertile women and those who are no longer capable of bearing offspring. It's as if we are put out to pasture and left to wander without purpose or value. Finding a way to absorb the realities of your changing body without also buying into all the limiting and, frankly, depressing attitudes our society holds about older women can be as perplexing as it is challenging. In fact, this may be a balancing act as taxing as the one many of us performed when we were working and raising kids and trying to "have a life" at the same time. Attempting to fulfill multiple roles taught us that the balance is never static. We were always in flux, trying to meet the constantly evolving needs of others. There was little time for us. Now that we're in our post-menopausal years, we are all faced with the task of creating equilibrium between honest acknowledgment and acceptance of the impact of aging on our bodies and a positive, encouraging sense of sexual self-esteem.

> I was told by my mother that at 34 there was no need for sex anymore. Once you stopped having children, there was no need for sex.
>
> —*Lydia, 55, Cheyenne, Wyoming*

What Really Happens: Your Sexual Physiology Beyond 50

By the time we've celebrated our 50th birthdays, it's assumed that we know it all when it comes to sex and how our bodies respond. Been there, done that—it's old hat. Yet the fact is that as women move beyond 50 we go through a transformation quite nearly as dramatic as that which occurs at adolescence. But there is no "birds and bees" lecture to teach us about what's happening.

When we talk with older women about our work, we are often bombarded with questions about the physical aspects of sexual aging.

"What is going on with my body?" "Will this lack of desire (or dull-ness of sensation or change in my response) continue, grow worse, get better?" Thirty-five percent of the women we surveyed declared that physical changes caused by hormonal changes are affecting their cur-rent level of sexual desire, and they continue to ask, "What's happen-ing to me, and what's going to happen ten years from now?'

When we all were approaching puberty, we needed to learn the basic facts of life; we needed some preparation for what was about to happen to our bodies. Few of us had parents who were comfortable talking with their children about sex. The information we found in books was generally presented in a cartoonish fashion or was so clinical that it made little sense to a kid. If you had an older sibling or friend, you might have gotten a rather imaginative version of sex education at best.

Then, around fifth or sixth grade, our elementary schools of-fered the "sex talk," causing giggles and wild speculation. Usually the girls went to the auditorium with their teacher (if she was a woman) or the school nurse, and the boys followed the coach or P.E. teacher to the gym. With all the weird feelings that come with adolescence, there was great curiosity and need for an explanation. A splotchy filmstrip, an introduction to feminine hygiene products, and a pamphlet titled *You're a Young Lady Now* put out by the com-pany that manufactured Tampax was usually the bulk of what we got, but at least it filled in a few gaps in our knowledge. Of course, the focus was all on reproduction. It was easy to get the impression that your body was about to turn into a baby-making factory and your job was to keep the production line from going into action until you had a wedding ring on your finger.

That may not have been the most helpful approach to sex educa-tion, but it was usually better than nothing. Today, however, the gap in our knowledge about the post-menopausal sexuality remains unfilled. You can certainly find lots of books about menopause it-self, but the issues of sexual desire and sexual self-esteem are rarely mentioned. Friends may be willing to joke around about how their bodies are starting to look like their mothers' or pass along the latest Viagra joke, but conversations about what normal aging does to the female anatomy or how an older woman maintains her sexual self-worth are rare indeed.

As so many of the women in our study told us, "Talking about sexual desire just wasn't done." Giggling, 55-year-old Ginny said, "Now we mainly just kid about it, we talk about spouse's lack of ability. One friend told me about taking testosterone and how that increased her desire, but that was unusual. We don't usually talk about that. Though we might tell jokes about Viagra. It's usually pretty light-hearted." Even women who have careers in health care are often just as much in the dark about the sexual changes that take place in aging female bodies as medically unsophisticated women.

> Women my age, my group of friends, we talk about it. We wouldn't talk about our intimacy, one-to-one personal sexual encounters with a partner, but we would talk very openly about changes in our bodies and "What do you think? Is this happening to you?" I valued that more than what I got in books.
>
> —*Scarlet, 60, Rapid City, South Dakota*

Talking with our health-care providers can be disappointing because many doctors have limited time for such a discussion or may be young enough to be our children or grandchildren. The fact is that during medical school and residencies, the vast majority of physicians—even obstetricians and gynecologists—have received very little education about sexuality in general, and next to none about sexuality in older adults. They are often uncomfortable with the notion that older people are curious about how to enhance their sexual lives.

But without the basic information about the normal process of aging and how it affects our sexual lives, we are left to our own imaginations. If we had a more complete appreciation for the natural process of sexual aging and understood how women's bodies are transformed, we could see our own sexuality in the softer light of the second half of life. The scale needs to be recalibrated, the words redefined. We need to match our internal vision of our bodies to our physical realities. Step 1 is learning about what actually happens. How does a normally aging, relatively healthy female body change sexually after menopause? Here are a few of the highlights:

1. **With menopause our ovaries become less responsive to stimulation by follicle-stimulating hormone (FSH) and luteinizing hormone (LH).** To try to compensate for the decreased response, the body produces more of these ovary-stimulating hormones for a time. The level of these hormones eventually decreases. The ovaries continue to produce small amounts of testosterone and some estrogen. The hormones produced by the pituitary gland also decrease. This reduction in hormones leads to a shut down of our reproductive capacity. Women who go through surgical menopause (hysterectomy) experience these same changes, though usually in a much more immediate and concentrated fashion. Our bodies are no longer in a state of preparation for pregnancy, and those areas that are most involved in reproduction begin to function differently.

2. **There is a reduction in blood flow to the pelvis.** Because of this, the pubic muscles lose tone. The Venus mound, or mons, loses plumpness and definition. This is one of those changes, along with the fact that our pubic hair thins, that is startling for many older women. At one of our discussion groups, Sandra, a woman in her mid-60s, remarked, "One day I was in the shower and I just looked

down at myself and realized my pubic hair was white and thin! I was horrified. I never thought about that happening." In fact, up to a third of menopausal and postmenopausal women in this culture experience general thinning of all their hair.

3. **The vagina goes through a real transformation.** It becomes shorter and narrower; secretions become scant and watery; the walls become less elastic, thinner, and less firm. The friction of intercourse or other penetration can cause them to bleed more easily than prior to menopause. The cervix may atrophy and flatten out to the wall of the vagina. Changes in the lining of the urethra and bladder can cause irritation and urinary frequency, urgency, and recurrent cystitis. There are changes in the levels of normal microorganisms in the vagina and in the pH level leading to an increased risk of vaginal yeast infections.

> The quality of my orgasms has changed—not as intense and requires more stimulation (vibrator) and lubrication (artificial)—not multi orgasmic anymore.
> —*Erica, 60, Wisconsin*

4. **Sexual arousal generally takes longer in post-menopausal women than in younger ones.** Vaginal wetness usually takes 1 to 3 minutes in women over 40, compared to 10 to 30 seconds for younger women. The external genital tissue decreases, and the clitoris shrinks in size, though it remains sensitive and capable of delivering sexual pleasure well into the ninth decade of life. In older women, the vagina may not lubricate, though this is not a universal experience.

Colette, now 85, had been celebate for several years following her husband's death. She recently reconnected with an old high-school flame and became sexually active again. "Before I became intimate, I sought the advice of a gynecologist who advised liberal use of lubrication. To my great surprise and the delight of my partner, artificial lubrication was not necessary."

5. **Sexual intercourse may become uncomfortable** for some women either because of decreased lubrication or the fact that the vagina is shorter and narrower and has decreased ability to expand during arousal and climax. The external genitals can become irritated by friction as well. The tissues of the labia majora and minora become less engorged than in younger women during sexual arousal. The uterus does not enlarge as much during arousal in women over 40, either. So the experience of intercourse and climax can feel quite different from how it felt in younger days.

6. **The breasts respond to sexual arousal differently in older women than in younger ones.** In women 51 to 60, the colored circular area around the nipple swells less during arousal than in younger women. The breasts of women over 60 seldom swell.

7. **Older women rarely experience sexual flushing with arousal.** In about half of women aged 41 to 50, sexual arousal is accompanied by a measleslike flush that spreads over the upper chest, neck, and face. This reddening occurs in only a little more than 10 percent of women aged 51 to 60. Women in the older age group are more likely to experience "hot flashes" than sexual flushes.

8. **There is evidence that women who do not have penetrative sex for 5 to 10 years after menopause, either through masturbation or intercourse, eventually have trouble with penetration.** We talked with a number of widows in the course of our research, and many of them had not had intercourse in several years. Several of the women in our study who became sexually active after a long hiatus overcame penetration difficulties without too much stress. For example, a 65-year-old widow from Phoenix told us,

"I was excited about starting a sexual relationship with a new man, but I was so surprised that our first encounter was so painful for me. I thought I must have some horrible sexual disorder. I was so worried I sought out a sex therapist. It only took one session with her to discover that I didn't have a disorder. All I needed was some honest conversation with my new guy and some lubricant for me."

The Hormone Question

The fact is, the physical effects of menopause are directly linked to our shifting hormones. There is no doubt that hormones are also major players in the complex experience of sexual desire. So it's easy to understand why the idea of replacing depleted hormones through HRT (hormone replacement therapy) is so appealing. If we could reverse or at least halt the aging process by keeping our hormones at youthful levels, wouldn't we all be happier? But when it comes to intervening medically to rebalance hormone levels that have been altered in menopause, older women are increasingly confused and frustrated by the conflicting information they receive.

As Holly, a 53-year-old bartender, said, "I think that hormone replacement therapy (HRT) is a loaded subject. I've been struck by how people are so opinionated and insist on telling others what's best for them rather than letting women make their own decisions." And Marianne, a grandmother of four who participated in a HRT clinical trial in her hometown of Philadelphia, was surprised by the effect that the hormones had on her unconscious sex life. "I filled out a questionnaire about quality of life before and after I was taking the prescribed medications. On the post-treatment questionnaire I wrote out that I was having sex dreams. I hadn't realized that before I started the trial I had stopped having them. I then realized I must be on HRT and not placebo."

Our research suggests that women often looked to HRT with the hope of revitalizing their sexual desire, but their experience was not consistently rewarding. Marilyn, a 69-year-old retired college professor from Berkeley, California, reported, "I did try HRT; however, the side effects were too painful for me to continue with it so I stopped. I then used soy supplements to alleviate hot flashes. That worked and I no longer use any supplements."

When we compared the women in our study who were currently taking hormone replacement therapy with those who are not, we found that those on HRT were significantly more likely to say that "sex is less enjoyable than it was in the past." And those women who had taken HRT in the past but have now stopped were the most likely to believe that in the next 10 years sex will be more enjoyable for them than it is today. Some women started taking HRT with a hope that things would improve for them sexually, but that didn't occur. After they stopped taking hormones, they looked forward to more sexual pleasure.

Another point of view is offered by the 47 percent of the women who responded to our survey who were currently taking some form of HRT and found that it had had a solidly beneficial influence on their sexual lives. Doris's doctor recommended she stop taking Premerin after she'd been on it for several years. "Too bad I can't take HRT any longer. It was great!"

"I am getting testosterone injections every three weeks, and that has helped with sexual desire," says Mavis, 52, from Memphis. The approach Mavis is taking, added testosterone, is one that is getting a lot of recent attention. We heard from a number of women who had experimented with it, and the reports were mixed. At the time of this writing, a type of testosterone designed to increase sexual desire in women has recently failed to get FDA (Food and Drug Administration) approval. The potential health risks—and benefits—from HRT make examination of the many other influences on sexual desire imperative before considering this treatment. (Please consult with your family physician or obstetrician-gynecologist, as new study results are frequently reported.)

Hormones may well be at the core of the our post-menopausal metamorphosis, but should we rush to stop their decline? The alterations in the contours of our bodies, the loss of muscle tone, the drying of the skin, and the tendency to form wrinkles and lose hair, to develop age spots and double chins—all these come with the new territory of life beyond 50. These types of changes may be inevitable, but are they necessarily to be lamented? Our attitudes and beliefs toward our aging bodies can leave us feeling appreciative of life's bounteous sensuality or resentful and angry over our lost youth.

The Body Image Struggle

That well-practiced critical eye we've so diligently trained on our less-than-perfect figures is ready to focus on our maturing bodies with devastating judgment. Our culture tends to equate a woman's worth with her sexual appeal, and that appeal is stereotypically defined in narrow, physical terms. Is there a mature woman in America today who hasn't felt the pressure to evaluate her body by the standard of deprivation set by the model Twiggy in the 1960s? You may not have bought into the thin-at-all-costs ideology completely—perhaps you were or are an athlete, or your support system encouraged robust health and enjoyment of food—

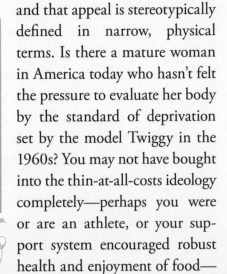

My sister and I might joke, but we are going to start getting serious about cosmetic surgery! My mother has had a lot of it, and we used to be very critical of her in the past, but now I would definitely consider it and I think it is all about my desirability.

—Ingrid, 63
Evergreen, Colorado

but it is unlikely that you were untouched by the tendency of our society to value the svelte over the Rubenesque.

When Prince Charles married Camilla Parker Boles in the spring of 2005, the media had a field day. They condemned Camilla for carrying on an affair with a married man and for being a home-wrecker. But her major sin, it is clear, is that she simply wasn't sexy—not in ways our society currently recognizes, and certainly not in relation to the youthful Diana. "Now that we have a real-life princess who is a woman of a certain age with liabilities…children, pets, an ex, a touch of jowls," wrote Daphne Merkin in *The New York Times Magazine*, March 6, 2005, "perhaps we are ready to re-examine what we mean when we use the term sexy." Unless we rede-fine sexuality in more broadly meaningful ways, we will remain stuck in the matron's closet.

Georgia, a stately 82-year-old from Maine, described what such a redefinition can do for you: "I have come to trust my body more than I used to. When I was anxious about my appearance, whether my husband desired me, whether I was going to have a satisfying sexual relationship, I was a lot more worried if my libido dropped. I am a lot easier now. I just do whatever comes naturally."

Often before they reach puberty girls are skilled at analyzing their bodies with a disparaging eye—to be painfully aware of their bulges and flab, to decry flat chests and flat butts, to wish for what they don't have. Many women talked with us about how their mothers or older relatives taught them to think of their bodies in negative ways.

"My mother never told me I was pretty. She loved me but was always pointing out my big hips or my unruly hair—saying boys aren't going to go for that. I think her main concern was that she was afraid I wouldn't find a husband," says Zoë, a 56-year-old Bud-dhist from California.

While we were young, we may have disliked our bodies in gen-eral, or were self-conscious about particular parts, but we had youth going for us at least. Now that our bodies are older, our critical selves can really have a heyday. Those women who were blessed with bodies that fit the youthful, sexy requirements may suffer even more as they observe the changes age brings. Carmen, a statuesque 54-year-old from Houston, said, "I've always thought I had a pretty good body. Lately, though, I've begun torturing myself about the way I look. My breasts are sagging, I've gained some weight, and now I think I have a chin waddle. I hate the way I look naked."

That exaggerated ideal we compare ourselves to is hard to avoid—she's on the cover of every magazine. And once we pass through the threshold and enter the world of the over 50, the comparison becomes almost comical. Our research suggests that there is a direct connection between how sexually appealing to others we believe ourselves to be and our own ability to experience sexual desire.

> I've kind of become accustomed to being without a sexual partner, and my sexual desire goes away. I've redirected my sexual energy towards my learning how to love myself and being happy with me. But sometimes the weather, especially springtime, brings it back. When all of the world starts waking up, so do I.
>
> —*Ellyn, 69, Kansas City, Missouri*

Melanie's story is also illustrative: "One thing that I have noticed is how my body image has changed lately. I never understood why women would put themselves down all the time. I was always very happy with the way I looked. In the last year, I am much more dissatisfied." Melanie, who recently turned 55, has been single all her life. She's had many lovers.

In answer to our question, "What kinds of things arouse an older woman's desire?" Corky, a 61-year-old massage therapist, answered, "Being desired by a man, feeling like you look good, feeling desirable. Some of it is feeling physically good about yourself and the way you look. I think that's attractive to men. If men find you attractive, it arouses your desire."

What happens then when you no longer believe you are attractive? Does this self-judgment lead inevitably to the end of your sexuality?

We learned many valuable lessons from women who have made the transition from youth to old age with grace and dignity without abandoning their sexual selves. The notion of taking care of their physical selves remained an important priority for them, but a significant shift had taken place. They talked about doing it for themselves now, not just to please their sexual partner or to be attractive to a man. And it isn't as much about appearance as it is about the pleasure of the sensual experience. And of course, self-care has myriad expressions. Tammy, a 52-year-old waitress from Idaho Falls, said, "My mother, who is in her 80s, told me she still sleeps without any clothes on, she likes the feel of the sheets on her body. She was sort of alluding to the fact that these feelings were kind of sexual…"

Redefining Sexy

"When I was young I knew a couple of women who were not mentors, per se, but women whom I felt were wholly sexy—women in their 80s at that point—and who emanated this real self-assuredness, who exuded a lot of sexuality, and I thought *Oh my gosh! They are so together,*" Lorraine, a 58-year-old cannery worker from Anchorage, told us. "It has nothing to do with even discussing anything about sexuality with them. This had to do with where they were with themselves, very grounded. I sensed a great sense of power and motherliness and warmth and kindness. As I become older I thought, *That is how I want to be.* They followed their own theme."

We were impressed with the fact that, no matter their age or their body type, when it comes to finding a path to self-acceptance, older women can't be pigeonholed. The avenue any one woman travels to reach a level of comfort with her sexuality will not necessarily work for someone else. Each woman's choice reflects her individual style.

Some women have resolved to change their bodies through plastic surgery. These women decided that as long as they were altering their physical persona for themselves, and not for others, a nip here and a tuck there could make all the difference in their self-esteem. Emma began writing poetry at 75 when she lost her third husband. Her blue eyes had begun to take on a milky glow, and her face was darkened with age spots. "I thought, *I'm not going to live like this. There's too much still to enjoy.* I got my boobs done, had the flab removed from my upper arms, and sanded those liver spots from my face. I was preparing myself for a new start. I'd always wanted to be a writer, and it was now or never. Then I decided that I couldn't be a writer and live in the South—you have to be born to that. I'm from New England, and I couldn't take the heat and humidity. I moved to the Northwest and I love the gray, soft, moist air. I walk whenever I can just to feel my body move." A good cup of coffee with new friends she's made at the retirement home, a hug from a companion, the voluptuous feel of poetry in her mouth as she reads aloud—all these sensuous experiences fill Emma's soul and connect her to her sexual self. She describes herself as "very much a woman in love with life." There is no doubt that this is one sexy lady.

Plastic surgery can enhance sexual self-esteem even at the end of life, as evidenced by Edith, a 55-year-old nurse from Indianapolis. "I once had a hospice patient who had breast implants. I went to see her the day before she died. She was naked in her bed, and she was so proud of her breast implants. And she said, 'Look at my body; it's a mess, but look at these breasts.' At first I did kind of a judgment, 'God, you're dying and all you're concerned about is your silicone breasts.' But after about 30 seconds, it was like, 'This is one incredible woman.'"

Other women we've encountered wouldn't think of going under a surgeon's scalpel. Instead, they have opted to flex their bodies on a regular basis and pay more attention to what they are putting into their mouths. Helen, a rosy-cheeked, pleasingly plump Nebraskan of Polish extraction, just celebrated her 75th birthday. She's been working out with weights at a gym near her riverside home for several years. More recently, she overcame her fear of water and enrolled in a water aerobics classes. With a twinkle in her eye, she told us, "A few years ago, I wouldn't have dreamt that I'd become a healthy water baby. I never had much time for exercise when my three kids were in school and my husband and I were struggling to make ends meet. You can see by my body that I've always enjoyed food, but since I joined the club, I have actually gained muscle tone and am a lot more flexible. My granddaughters get a kick out of playing in the kiddy pool while I push my foam barbell. Not only do I feel better physically, I'm showing them that exercise is something even old ladies can do."

Rather than altering their physical selves, a large percentage of women have focused on amending their long-held attitudes toward their bodies. They have begun to revel in their appearance. Frances, a 70-year-old retiree currently living in Louisiana, told us, "I am very busty, more than a double-D my whole life. And it has been a problem for me my whole life. My mother would buy me bras, spending so much time trying to make me look smaller. Instead of accepting them I have always been fighting them. I even went to a doctor about it...what he told me he had to do was to take off the nipples when they do the operation (breast reduction) and then they put the nipples back and then the nipples never have sensation. And that idea has always been a real turn-off for me. So it has come to the point where I have made peace with who I am."

Another woman, 53-year-old Juanita, had a slightly different take. "As we age, I think we just naturally slow down. I think it is common for a lot of women that if they don't feel sexy in themselves they don't feel attractive. I guess that I understand that, but I don't feel that way. I don't feel unattractive or undesirable or unsexual because I don't have the same sexual desires. I know I am a beautiful woman. And that I can still be beautiful, whether I am having sex or not. It is not how often I am having sex that makes me beautiful."

Still other women are concentrating on enjoying newfound sensuality rather than focusing on their external appearance. For example, Monica, a 62-year-old former assembly line worker, said, "I think about walking through the woods in Wisconsin, or being in a cabin or in front of a fireplace, you know...some physical thing. I am not a person to go out dancing or get a sexy dress on. I am much more laid back; I find a lot more intimacy in nature and quiet spaces, like my garden."

Paying attention to their bodies is a new experience for some older women. Many have told us that a little personal pampering elevates their spirits and satisfies their sensual needs. Irene, a 52-year-old mother of two teenage sons still living at home, told us how self-care improved her mind-set. "I go get a massage and a facial; I do something that is tactile for me. I sense that if I go into this self-care, whether it's buying new cosmetics or something else satisfying, I don't consciously notice [that my sexual desire is less]. I just feel attractive and it gives me a boost."

Women are revising the meaning of sexuality to fit the second half of life. Consider 95-year-old Rosalyn, who lives in a retirement home in Baton Rouge and describes herself as a real flirt. "I am legally blind, but my body is great. I could still be out there dancing if I could see better!" Rosalyn is a late-life artist who gives expression to her creative imagination by making wild and wonderful hats.

Her life is full of contact with men, all of whom she appreciates. "On Sunday morning I go to church and oh my, guys, they all run over to me and kiss me, and hug me. It is just the touching, the contact that makes me very happy. I just want to hold their hand and giggle and laugh with them and dance."

It may well be time to readjust your "sexiness scale" and begin to value your aging body. Finding ways to accept the body you've been dealt today and see past self-described imperfections is an ongoing project. You may find it helpful to start by doing an inventory of the attitudes you are carrying around in your head that may limit your ability to make this readjustment.

Your Personal Definitions of Sexy

The following questions are designed to help you identify your personal beliefs and attitudes about sexiness in older women.

Answer the following questions:

1. What did your mother (grandmother, or other older woman) teach you (directly or indirectly) about sexiness and aging?

2. How have cultural (society/media/religion) portrayals of older women and sexiness affected you?

3. What is your image of a sexually vibrant older woman?

Now take a moment to think about how realistic and optimistic your attitudes are. Consider how Hattie, a 60-year-old painter who lives and works in Las Vegas, has revised her thinking. "There was a woman I didn't even know, but she had a beautiful body and I was sad that my body wasn't beautiful like that woman's body. That was a reality check for me. But I know there are women in the arts who are revered and still work up into their 80s. To me, that's what really keeps me going. It doesn't matter what I look like, how wonderful I perform at parties, I can still keep making art—that's coming from within me. That's my source of energy and self-confidence."

If you want to work on developing a more appreciative stance toward your aging body, here are a few suggestions and some questions for you to ponder.

1. Revise how you speak about your own body and those of other older women. Words are amazingly powerful tools when it comes to maintaining or changing attitudes. Christine, who is 63 and lives in Denver, told us, "When my friends and I get together lately we're always complaining about something with our bodies. I'm getting so fat, or I am so wrinkled, or my skin is so dry. It's a downer." Imagine how different the atmosphere around Christine and her friends would be if they made a point of talking about their bodies in positive terms. It can be tough to resist the pull to focus on the negative, but giving yourself credit for your strengths has many emotional benefits.

Esther, a widow in her mid-70s, proudly described how she and her friends bolster one another's self-confidence with frequent compliments. "When I get together with my girlfriends I always feel better. We are constantly telling each other 'you look so nice today' or 'you lost some weight, it's good for you.' It's important to hear that sort of thing, otherwise you kind of get down on yourself. I have good friends."

Scan the Sunday newspaper or the weekly newsmagazines for disparaging comments and descriptions of older women's bodies. Once you become aware of how ubiquitous this kind of criticism is, you can begin to reject it. You may even want to write a letter to the editor challenging the images! If we each begin with our own words, our own voices, and our own attitudes, we can change our culture. Rather than comparing yourself in negative ways, you can

The Sensuality of Music

Many women equate music with sensuality, and certain songs or artists trigger their desire. Women who grew up in the 1940s talked about how a tune from Frank Sinatra could stimulate all kinds of sexy feelings. Women who grew up going to sock hops in their high school gyms kept talking about Johnny Mathis and Elvis's music and how their songs continue to affect their moods today.

A number of black women cited the sultry voices of men such as Nat King Cole, Luther Vandross, and Barry White as turn-ons. For many women, Revel's "Bolero" was at the top of their hit parade; for others it was Pacabel's "Canon in D." One Hispanic woman told us, "Latin beats—the rhumba, the samba, and the tango—get me gyrating and my blood flowing."

be a mirror for other women—you can reflect their beauty and help them see it. Consider getting some of your women friends together for an evening of body positive talk. It's a challenge for all of us, so give yourselves credit for any forward movement.

2. **Appreciate your sensuality and reframe your responsiveness.** There are benefits that come with a body that is slowing down. Attend to your internal sensations rather than focusing on how others see you. This shift can connect you to new delights as you learn how your mature body sings its own songs. Wrinkles and extra flab provide more surface area for tactile pleasure; our drooping contours and rounded shape may help us to move differently in the world.

Noreen, a 63-year-old Texan with a contagious twang and blue eyes that match the cornflowers in her yard, says, "One of things I love most about water aerobics is stepping down the stairs into the pool and feeling the water swirling around my entire body and caressing my limbs. It's the best way for me to start my day."

Think about which smells and music appeal to you. Which ones are turn-offs? What colors and textures do you like? Is velvet your favorite fabric, or is chiffon the one that evokes positive memories of an unforgettable prom night? What about the weather? Do the rain and mist offer more appeal and comfort for you, or are you a sun worshipper albeit with lots of sunscreen?

The relationship between food and sensuality for women is complex. For many of us, food has become a challenge that defies our best intentions. If we give in to the lure of our appetites, we struggle with the consequence of added weight, which we equate with less sexual appeal. On the other hand, eating can be a richly sensual experience for many older women. There are ties between certain foods or the circumstances when foods are eaten and the sensation of the body responding to pleasure. We've asked women about foods that stirred up their desire. Their tastes vary widely, but there was a consensus about the most sensuous (and now considered to have definite health benefits) food: chocolate. Wine and champagne, spicy foods, succulent foods, gooey foods were also near the top of the list. At one discussion group, a woman demonstrated the way juicy foods dripped down her arms, enhancing both her desire and her delight. When asked his take on the relationship between desire and food, noted Seattle chef and author Tom Douglas told us, "Oh, yeah, there's really something to this, but for women, it's not oysters!"

> Tequila makes me want to take my clothes off—my partner and I both enjoy fish, sushi and sashimi a lot.
>
> —*Barbara, 53*
> *Big Sur, California*

3. **Take good care of yourself.** Though you may still be actively involved in a pressured career or find yourself raising grandchildren,

it is time to readjust your focus
and frame yourself at the center.
Eighty-two-year-old Flo told us
to remember that "the music of
life isn't over until the musicians
have packed up their instruments
and left. If you want to keep on
playing in the band, wear lipstick. Pay attention to your body.
Stay attractive if only for yourself
and the world in general."

Many women beyond 50
have yet to learn to spoil them-

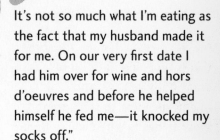

> It's not so much what I'm eating as
> the fact that my husband made it
> for me. On our very first date I
> had him over for wine and hors
> d'oeuvres and before he helped
> himself he fed me—it knocked my
> socks off."
>
> —*Rayanne, 56*
> **Wilmington, North Carolina**

selves. Sure, you may have tried the candles and bubble bath route
once or twice a year or taken a new spa up on its two-for-one massage offer. But after years of telling yourself, "I need to save my
money to buy a new washing machine" rather than spending cash
on a pedicure, it is past the time to reset the dial. Self-care revital-
izes your soul and reduces your stress. Set aside some time just for
you. It can help you become more sensually aware. It may even help
you overcome petty jealousy and fears about your aging body.

Regardless of whether you're partnered or not, whether your
desire is blazing or nil, whether your sexual self-esteem is surging or
it needs a tune-up, you can treat your body as a sexual object—sexy
and sensuous to you. You can propel yourself down the path of redefining sexy by buying a new perfume or a new moisturizer, wearing the colors you like, taking a dance or Pilates class, skipping that
third chocolate cookie in lieu of a vitamin pill, or even giving yourself permission to indulge in your favorite sensual food.

When groups of post-menopausal women get together, the talk often leads to complaints of "back fat" and expanding waistlines.

Practicing Self-Care

Ask yourself: "What are the three things I'm going to do to take care of my body as I age, and exactly when I am going to start doing these things?" When you've done each one, evaluate it—how did it make you feel? If your experience was positive, make another date with yourself; let it become a habit.

They may jokingly discuss the possibility of getting a group discount from a plastic surgeon for reductions of their now-pendulous 38 DDDs, or empathize over their flabby upper arms and deepening crow's feet. This type of self-effacing, negative talk comes naturally to women brought up to focus on their physical flaws. We learn to label as "bad" any attributes that distinguish our body from that of the Mattel figurine or our personal Barbie stand-in. Our culture has taught us that even if we do like the way we look, we certainly aren't supposed to call attention to our strengths. This failure to appreciate our own bodies combined with our tendency to equate sexual appeal with youth and beauty leave us especially vulnerable to discouragement when we reach the beyond-50 years.

But once we understand what is really happening to our bodies as we age and what we can expect physiologically, we are better prepared to examine our attitudes toward our aging sexual selves. By realistically redefining the meaning of *sexy*, by rejecting the physical scale by which our culture has weighed your worth, by learning to pamper yourself and to appreciate your sensuality, you can foster your sexual self-confidence and appreciate the power and the beauty of being an older woman.

Together mature women can begin to reshape our society's dismissive judgment of us. Rosalyn, a retired high school counselor, is a woman whose body has softened with age, yet she radiates charm and sexual vibrancy. She embodies a dynamism, sensuality, and creativity that inspire those around her. Her friend Mary says, "At 70, Rosalyn is a very vital, energetic woman. Even though she doesn't have a partner, I see her as attractive in all ways. Sexuality is just part of it. My goal is to be like my friend and age gracefully."

Truth #3

Less Can Be More After 50

How to Find Joy When Sexual Desire Ebbs

In an elegant townhouse adorned with family photos and mementos, 12 older women eyed each other apprehensively as they sat on chairs and sofas drinking coffee. "Sexual desire? I'd rather be picking apples." Dorothy's candid statement elicited hoots of laughter and murmurs of agreement from the women. The hostess, Jane, owner of a local travel agency, had invited a number of colleagues and friends to join in a discussion of sexual desire and aging led by the authors. Dorothy is an outspoken, vivacious 65-year-old social worker who had initially responded to Jane's invitation with a dismissive "Oh, you don't want me. My sexual desire dried up years ago." But she changed her mind when Jane asked her if her lack of desire was troubling.

> My desire is less intense now. I do not define sexual desire as simply wanting to have sex. It includes deep joys, emotional pleasures, and intimate contact whether physical, spiritual, or emotional.
>
> —*Selma, 55, Fort Worth, Texas*

The reality was that in the last eight years or so, Dorothy's desire had melted away. There was no abrupt shutting down, just a gradual waning. At first, she was a bit alarmed. What effect would this change have on her intimate life? After all, she and her second husband Brad had only been married for five years. She had worried that he'd be pretty upset. In her first marriage to Joel, she'd attributed any drop in her ardor to the problems they were having. But this new relationship was just the opposite of her previous one. Money wasn't too much of an issue, and neither was communication. She and Brad took long, ambling walks, wandering hand in hand through the pasture on their farm. They debated which varieties of heirloom tomatoes to plant and discovered early on that they both liked salt and pepper on their cantaloupe. Knowing she wanted to keep this partnership for life, she'd taken a number of deep breaths and talked to him about her sexual feelings. Gently, Dorothy let Brad know that her desire had evaporated; it was just gone. She told him she didn't know if it would be coming back, but for the foreseeable future, she was quite content with companionship and hugs. Brad's response was surprisingly positive, and they'd settled into a comfortable, relaxed routine. Now, for the first time, Dorothy found she wanted to openly acknowledge that tending her small apple orchard was honestly more of a draw for her these days than the idea of a sexual encounter. She thought perhaps that describing her situation would be helpful to someone else in the room. In fact, her frank admission did not reveal any pain or regret. "I'm just fine with it. My life is very full, and my husband and I are quite satisfied."

Is Low Desire Really a Dysfunction?

It's commonly believed that diminishing desire in the older woman is an inevitable and depressing reality of aging. But sometimes "common knowledge" is flat wrong. The majority of women do

experience a decrease in their sexual desire once they are past menopause, but contrary to popular opinion, many do not find this shift
depressing. True, the quest to regain lost libido is a frustrating obsession for many older women, and we do often hear the plaintive
plea, "How do I get it back?" But this isn't the universal concern
that the Western media and pharmaceutical industry would have us
believe it is.

Powered by their investors and their bottom-line-driven CEOs,
the drug companies have focused on those women who are dismayed by their lagging libido. They have helped to reinforce the
myth that feeling youthful lustiness is what all older women want.
Until recently, a number of pharmaceutical companies touted the
benefits of hormone replacement therapy (HRT) as a panacea for
rejuvenating flagging desire.

Research has demonstrated that HRT may cause more harm
than good if taken for long periods of time or if a woman's family
history is rife with breast cancer and heart problems. Now drug
companies, researchers, doctors, and even some sexologists are for-
saking a HRT approach and are instead asking, "Where is the
Viagra for women?" Millions of dollars are being spent to answer
this question.

Women with low desire are told they have a problem that needs
to be fixed. Magazines, TV shows, and medical trade journals keep
hyping an article about the 1999 National Health and Social Life
Survey that appeared in the *Journal of the American Medical Association* written by sociologist Dr. Edward Laumann and colleagues.
The article reported that up to 43 percent of women suffer from
some kind of problem with sex. There is even a new disease category
called "sexual interest disorder." Canadian sexologist Dr. Rosemary
Basson, along with other pharmaceutical industry–funded researchers, suggests that one-third of all women may suffer from this disorder. Brian Deer, writing in *The London Sunday Times Magazine* on
September 28, 2003, quotes Dr. Basson: "If a woman has no interest

in sex, it's a disorder because it's out of line with the expected situation, and the range that seems to be normal." This may apply to the pre-menopausal crowd, but for women beyond 50, we've found that the range of normal is broad enough to include levels of desire that could be categorized as "gone."

Once low desire is classified as a medical malady, successful treatment requires visits to the doctor. And because doctors are in the business of fixing problems, they naturally reach for their prescription pad at the first mention of diminished sexual desire, not fully understanding that for many women, a decline in desire may well be in the normal range. Hurried and weary, physicians offer up medicine that may actually create additional problems. For example, Jamie, now in her mid-50s, had a hysterectomy at age 40. A single woman with several sexual partners, Jamie had been on estrogen since her surgery. After the Women's Health Initiative research study widely publicized its findings on the possible dangers of hormone replacement therapy, her doctor told her: "I just don't think you are

a candidate for estrogen. Let's try something else." So she put Jamie on Effexor (an antidepressant), and it had the effect of absolutely turning off her libido.

When it comes to offering treatments for this questionable problem, many options are available. Lately, there has been much talk about marketing a testosterone pill that would enhance sexual desire in women. The pharmaceutical companies are panting over the possibilities of developing one, but to date, no FDA approved magic remedy

Sleep Deprivation

A woman went to see her physician and said, "I've got a big problem, doctor. Every time we're in bed and my husband climaxes, he lets out this ear-splitting yell."

"My dear, said the doctor, "that's completely natural. I don't see what the problem is."

"The problem is," she said, "it wakes me up."

has reached the market. The FDA says more research is needed before it can be brought forward.

Bio-identical hormone treatments are yet another approach touted as the miracle cure for diminished desire in all older women. These are plant-based or "natural" hormones designed to be identical to the hormones produced by the human body. Many women feel that they are safer and perhaps even more effective than traditional hormone replacement therapy. But other women say, "I'm not sure I would take something like Viagra, or seek out a pharmacy that compounds bio-identical hormones or use a testosterone patch if it was available. Do I really need all this?"

Such a perspective is offered by Cindy, a 55-year-old nurse living in the Northeast, who says: "Sexual desire is just not that important to me. My husband and I have sex one time per month, and that is exactly as I like it. I don't consider it important in terms of my health and well-being. You know, you hear about the development of a Viagra for women and people who want more desire. I think I could work it up if I wanted to, but I don't care if I don't have it. I realize that my desire has decreased a lot. It doesn't concern me. If my husband wants to have intercourse, I might have a smidgen of desire. I will have sex if I feel like it. But if I don't, I won't. I don't object to it, but it is basically for him. I have found a lot of things that I do that I enjoy doing, and sexual desire just doesn't come into play. I enjoy quilting, going to the movies, and sewing."

Are we mature women truly aching to restore adolescent cravings to our lives? Is lower libido in the older woman really a new disease of stratospheric proportions or only another distortion in a long line of inaccuracies about women's sexuality? Is low sexual interest a cause for alarm, or does this spin have more to do with rewarding drug company stockholders than with helping women? Psychologist Leonore Tiefer and others suggest that it is time for a new view of women's sexuality. We couldn't agree more. Pharmaceutical product development of a "pink Viagra," culturally induced sexual anxieties, traditional sex education models describing women's sexual response cycles, and plain old greed have combined to obscure what older women are honestly experiencing. Although some women do mourn the loss of desire and yearn to restore it, our research suggests that for a large percentage of mature

> I was a *very* sexual person throughout my life…I was promiscuous, and luckily I didn't catch any horrible diseases. Sex permeated my thoughts…Suddenly, I turned 50 and I stopped having those thoughts.
> —*Sylvia, 63, Chicago*

women, diminished desire does *not* interfere with their zest for life, their feeling toward their partners, or their sexual self-esteem. Afterall, if more then 50 percent of women experience a decrease in desire, isn't that the norm?

The Truth About Low Sexual Desire

The more we listen to voices from women around the country, the more aware we are that the positive aspects of waning sexual desire in women beyond 50 has gotten a short shrift. In fact, Dorothy's declaration that she was not distressed by her decreased desire mirrors what many older women throughout America—suburbanites and ranchers; professional women and retirees; lesbians, bisexuals, and heterosexuals; women in long-term relationships; single women and divorcees; white women, black women, and Latinas—have told us: their sexual desire has faded, and that's okay with them. Women who are content with this shift accept that their desire will continue to ebb and flow as they age. They appreciate this as a natural result of aging and recognize that there are many things that influence it.

A decline in desire is generally the result of a confluence of factors including not only the physical and relational, but the emotional and even spiritual aspects of a woman's life as well. For example, 61-year-old Nannette from Peoria, Illinois, wrote to us, "Any feelings of desire depend so much on the balance I have in my life at any given day (if I feel good about myself or bad)."

We asked women to name the factors they felt had had a negative effect on their sexual desire since they had turned 50. Their own critical attitudes about how their bodies had changed, disruptions in sleep patterns and consequent fatigue, a boring sexual routine, or lack of a sexual partner were among the more prominent factors women listed. They also mentioned that "the blues" had caused their desire to flag, as did the loss of a spouse. Loretta, a reserved septuagenarian, said, "I have had less desire partially because of health, some because of my age, and some maybe because of my partner not being as romantic as he could be."

> Is candlelight a color that heightens desire? If so, hide the matches and turn up the lights.
>
> —*Ellen, 58, New Haven, Connecticut*

Filling all the roles that older women take on in their lives is taxing. In fact, 40 percent of women said fatigue chilled their desire. And the higher their income level, the more likely were women to mention that fatigue was a factor negatively affecting their cravings. Anita, a self-assured working mother of four in her early 50s who attended one of our discussion groups said, "Come on girls, wouldn't you just rather get a good night's sleep?"

And there may be something about turning 60. Sixty percent of women in their 60s reported that their desire was less than it used to be—more than women in any other decade beyond 50. Joanne, a colorful 68-year-old real estate agent from Los Angeles, told us, "I still consider myself a woman with passion, just not sexual desire at this time in my life. Sex is an area of my life I've let go of. A good romp in the hay is something no longer important to me as a woman."

Most women in our study mentioned that a combination of factors contributed to their diminished desire. The overall picture is a montage of influences that overlap and interrelate. Women who have had only one sexual partner in their lifetime are more likely than women who have had between two and twenty partners to say that their sexual desire had decreased. Coretta, a newly retired nurse, told us that she'd been looking forward to retirement because she thought it might allow her and her husband, who was the only man she'd ever slept with, a chance to reach a level of intimacy they hadn't experienced in years. "I do have desires and ideas towards having more sexual activities with my partner, but I don't have the follow-through. Something about the patterns that my partner and I have fallen into through the years turns me off." With a twinkle in her deep-set brown eyes, Charlene, a caterer from Cleveland who has been married for thirty years, whispered, "If you feed them really good, then they'll just want to go to sleep."

An Unspoken Truth

Women who live on the East Coast were more likely than those who lived in the South or on the West Coast to mention that fatigue had negatively influenced their sexual desire.

More than 51 percent of women said body image is the biggest single factor that contributes to decreased desire. Because this issue is so significant, we've dedicated an entire chapter to exploring it (see Chapter 2). Marjorie, in her late 50s and married for many years, told us, "Since my weight gain, I'm afraid of rejection and don't like to be touched or encouraged to be sexual. Rejection is always present."

Although 31 percent of women said they simply did not know

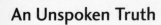

An Unspoken Truth

Married women are more likely
than their unmarried counterparts
to note that their sexual desire is
less than it used to be.

or refused to share with us what
factors were possibly affecting
their current level of sexual desire, many women reported that
their relationship status was a big
negative, one that contributed to
a decrease in desire. In fact, Le-
anne, a 56-year-old high-school
teacher from Los Angeles, said,
"As a younger woman, I was in-
credibly active sexually, having slept with over 75 men and some
women too. Much of the demise of my sexual desire I believe has to
do with being married."

At 69, Faith has been married to Roger for 40 years. Roger had
a demanding, high-level job in international business that required
him to be away from home for long stretches. Faith spent the early
years of their marriage raising their three kids, mostly on her own,
and awaiting Roger's homecomings with her sexual appetite at
high pitch. Once their children were grown and Faith had more
free time, she began a new career. The mounting energy and enthusiasm she felt for her work seemed to parallel her declining sexual
desire. "Creativity has replaced sex. I spend much time at the computer writing. I have my own publishing company and have written and published two books since I turned 60. The sexual and
emotional highs so extreme and prevalent when my husband was
traveling a lot have been replaced by an abiding love and the security of knowing that he's here for me, just as I am here for him."

Women who are widowed, divorced, dating, or not currently in
a relationship commented that not having a partner has caused a
significant change in their sexual desire. Megan, a 55-year-old divorced cosmetologist from Alabama, said, "I haven't been sexually
active in the last couple of years, and I don't really care that my desire is low. I met a man a few months ago and there was initially a

magnetic kind of attraction. But then about the third time I saw him I wasn't really sure any more. I don't think I talked myself out of it...I don't know why I am that ambivalent about it. Maybe I just don't want to rearrange my life."

The financial realities of widowhood and divorce also play a significant role in determining how a woman might rate her level of desire. Women whose annual income is less than $40,000 are more likely than their wealthier counterparts to identify the lack of a partner as affecting their level of sexual desire. And the higher the household income, the more likely a woman is to say that her sexual desire is less than it used to be.

An Unspoken Truth

Nearly 30 percent of women who had lower desire told us that at this point their sex life was mind-numbing, dreary, and lackluster. "Sex is fine and exciting when it is new. I feel it can last for three years—whether it be with your husband or a new relationship. Children take away the fire," says Gail, a 55-year-old divorced, mother of three adult children from Morgantown, West Virginia.

Genevieve, who is 58, told us that her and her husband Greg's yearly income is well over $160,000 a year. "I'm not interested in partner sex at all any more. Our marriage is okay; we've been married 31 years. We're not real tight or really lovey or anything like that, but I think we're fairly committed to staying together."

Perhaps these statistics reflect the fact that women with more money consider their sexual options from a different vantage point than those who are more focused on paying for their prescriptions and buying food. Without a sexual partner, who presumably might contribute to the financial health of the household, a woman's sexual desire may take a backseat to financial security. It be may be especially difficult for an older woman living alone on a meager, fixed Social Security income to even recognize her cravings.

The monetary consequences of partner loss are not always the cause of the greatest disruption in a woman's sexual self-esteem and desire, however. Sixty-year-old Natalie had a different kind of challenge in her marriage but has found paths to resolution: "About five years ago my husband told me he was gay. And that has changed a lot of my attitude toward my need for sex. At first I was very angry...for being lied to, for [his] using me as a sexual partner while he was having relationships with other men. So there was a lot of anger, and I turned myself off for a long time. I wondered whether I even wanted a sexual partner, but I am not willing to go outside the marriage to have it. I have never had multiple partners, and I wasn't about to start doing that at 55. I went through a lot of counseling over this, and the counselors helped me see that this wasn't about me, and there is nothing wrong with me. I've redirected my sexual energy. I am very social and outgoing. I have a lot of friends, I work hard, and I love my work. I garden, and I have done retreat work and focused on my spirituality."

An Unspoken Truth

Sixteen percent of women cited loss of a partner as having put a damper on their desire. "Since my husband died, my desire has faded away," says Ethel, 75, from Provo, Utah.

Delightful for Many, Depressing for a Few

Whether the primary forces that result in dwindling desire are age, relationship factors, body image, finances, fatigue, general health, or a combination of all these, the result can be a source of sadness and irritation or a cause for celebration. For many of the women in our study, the benefits over-shadow the negatives. Women are finding delight in myriad pleasurable activities in spite of, or perhaps due to, sexual desire that has gone out to sea.

Sylvia, a stunning woman in her early 60s who lives in Chicago with her husband of two years, suggests that lower desire has its pluses. A practi-

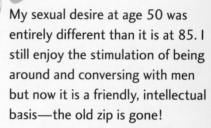

My sexual desire at age 50 was entirely different than it is at 85. I still enjoy the stimulation of being around and conversing with men but now it is a friendly, intellectual basis—the old zip is gone!

—*Grace, a thrice-married widow*
Valley Forge, Pennsylvania

cal, well-traveled woman, her body language conveys competence and self-awareness. When asked about her sexual history, Sylvia revealed that she had had well over a hundred lovers in her life. But when she talked about her husband, it was with the giddy pride of a new wife. "I never expected to be committed to one person, especially not at this late date. But he is just a wonderful, funny, sexy guy, and we really love each other. That's why my lack of desire—which came on just after my 50th birthday—has sur-prised me so much. At first it was disconcerting, because for the longest time sexual desire was such a major part of my life, and then suddenly it was gone."

Sylvia initially responded to this abrupt change in her libido by searching for a magic pill. She tried numerous remedies to help her regain her familiar high level of desire, but to no avail. Gradually, she began to recognize that life without the old sexual cravings had a lot of benefits. "The biggest thing about not thinking about sex anymore is that I can devote myself to my creative outlets. I can fo-cus better without the desire. I have become a much more creative photographer. I think more about where I can take my next great photograph. In a sense, it's why I didn't have my creative focus ear-lier. I used to have this insatiable sexual appetite. But now it's gone. Now my desire is to be wherever there is beauty. Photography has

An Unspoken Truth

Younger women (50 to 59) were significantly more likely than their older counterparts to say, "Sex is not as enjoyable for me now."

always been in my life, but the focus is so much stronger...and I know that is really what I want to be doing. My husband and I have a very loving relationship. It's just not a big deal for him that we don't have sex too often. My work is selling well. I have a website. I am doing exactly what I want to be doing."

As many women have told us, emotional needs and even relationship needs can be met without the sex act itself. Their stories represent one of the most encouraging findings that our study yielded: for scores of women, life has superseded sexual desire. Many described having very full, exciting, creative lives without having any sexual desire, or sexual activity, for that matter.

We've discovered that post-menopausal women's diminished desire is not a reason to panic, nor is it a dysfunction that needs to be fixed. For women with optimistic expectations, and those who are coming to the realization that they are not oddities, shifts in sexual desire can open the door to new avenues of excitement.

Imagine a future in which vibrant, imaginative women beyond 50 embrace their newfound freedom from the demands of their libidos, in which the post-menopausal years are anticipated as vistas filled with new options, in which mature women feel surging self-esteem right along with their hot flashes. Whether they are 55 or 68 or 90, women with a lower sex drive and those who modulate their desire to match their partner's do not necessarily have poor sexual self-esteem. Many respect and honor their own level of sexual desire, regardless of intensity—and their sexual self-confidence is alive and quite robust.

Dorothy, Sylvia, Natalie, and Faith have each taken different paths in dealing with her diminished desire. Their life circumstances have challenged them in different ways, yet like the scores of women from around the country with whom we have spoken, the process of adapting to their changed sexual appetites has had a positive outcome. Rather than grieving the loss of her sexual desire, Dorothy has been able to embrace this shift as a normal part of aging for her. She has been able to move forward in the context of her relationship without making significant changes in her behavior or her interests.

For Sylvia, having been an extremely sexually focused woman for most of her life, the abrupt drop in her desire came as a shock. She explored a variety of treatment options and considered a wide range of remedies before she was ready to accept her changed status. After a period of grieving, she discovered a new satisfaction through her creative endeavors.

Natalie's situation caused her a lot of pain and grief. It took her years to heal the wounds to her sexual self-esteem caused by her husband's revelation that he was gay. Her sexual desire plummeted, but she saw that alteration as an asset because her priority was self-protection. Eventually, she was able to make a conscious choice to redirect her passion toward personally fulfilling activities and away from sexual intimacy.

As Faith has aged, love and security have been elevated on her priority list. In the context of her long-term marriage, fewer highs and lows in desire have led to increased stability. She has found that though her physical ardor has diminished, her emotional connection with her husband has deepened.

These women, like so many others, have experienced confusion, heartache, and fear as they faced the reality of sexual desire in the years beyond 50. Yet they have discovered the surprising truth that diminished desire can

> I am currently asexual and very happy about it! I am able to see things in a different way and devote more time to previously neglected areas of my life.
>
> —*Laura, 58, librarian, Midlands, Texas*

pave the way for unexpected joys. There are parts of all of us that hide in the background during our youth and early middle age when sexual fervor and reproductive zeal commands center stage. Perhaps it is only after that curtain has dropped that we have the opportunity to appreciate other, previously less insistent, passions. As these women's stories reveal, acceptance of diminished sexual desire is not only possible, it can be downright joyful. All that is required is your willingness to break away from the restraints of culturally determined, well-worn habits and the flexibility to adopt an optimistic attitude. By exploring territory that is new to you, you may tease some shy talent out into the daylight. Without the need to fulfill intense sexual cravings, there is now time and energy for you to invest in yourself. Rather than allowing your sexual self-esteem to be limited by cultural stereotypes or the level of your sexual desire, you can nurture it by daring to reclaim your personal power, poise, and assurance.

Ten Other Avenues to Finding Fulfillment

If your desire has begun to ebb and the little voice within is trying hard to overcome blaring messages telling you "You must stay sexually active!", if sex is not the turn-on it once was for you, and your vaginal juices seem to be evaporating rather than flowing, then perhaps you're ready for a journey that takes you in a new direction. Consider the various paths taken by women like yourself. A little stroll down one or more of these many avenues of possibility may be just the ticket to finding your joy.

1. Main Street

As younger women, many of us were constantly overwhelmed. We had unrelenting obligations, careers to manage, and husbands or partners to satisfy. Finding quiet time to just enjoy our families has been a challenge. One of the many rewards of being older is the opportunity to simplify our lives and appreciate the joys of hearth and home, family and friends. "The energy that used to express itself as sexual lustiness is moving in a different direction," says Nancy, 62, from Springfield, Illinois. "I'm putting my energy into other things. Now that energy and the kind of relationships that I seek are more sensual than sexual. I have always had strong women friendships. But now we kiss and hug more; even with my friends' grandchildren and their children—I kiss and hug them—I like that. My animal creatures, my pets, my dogs, my cats, I touch them more. These seem to give me more pleasure on a daily basis, whether or not I have that tingle and burn in the erotic sense."

2. Wall Street

Money doesn't buy happiness, but financial security does play a big role in self-confidence. If you have avoided dealing with investments or even balancing your checkbook up to this point, you may discover that it can be quite empowering to take control of your finances. "Perhaps the joy I feel in managing my finances stems from being a scared, young, single mom once," says Wanda, 69, from Hartford, Connecticut. "I had no one to fall back on and had to make my own way. Now that I'm semi-retired, I've really gotten involved in managing my money. It's not that I don't trust a financial adviser; I just think it's great fun to see if I can beat the stock market averages on a regular basis."

3. Marathon Boulevard

Endorphins—those naturally occurring neurotransmitters that have pain-relieving properties similar to morphine—can produce euphoric feelings, stifle your appetite, and even release sex hormones. This experience is called a "runner's high," but you can enjoy a mild version of it after a water aerobics class or even a brisk walk. Says Pearl, age 58, from Phoenix: "I play a lot of tennis. In addition, I am at the gym four mornings a week. I swim, take step aerobics, take yoga classes. It's like a drug for me. And it's all healthy. And two of my friends who are in their 60s have taken up auto racing. They say it's a real rush!"

4. Broadway

Ever fantasized about seeing your name in lights? Although we may bemoan the limited roles available for older women in Hollywood, in truth, the opportunities are growing for women of any age in the arts. This may be the perfect time to explore your long-dormant interest in pottery or take up playing the piano. We talked with women in their 60s who were tap dancing for the first time, and others in their 80s who were writing their memoirs. At 54, Joan, who lives in Ames, Iowa, has discovered a new source of satisfaction: "I came off a real hard-science background—nursing—and I think that the arts give me the arena of everything that I really enjoy—color, textures, rhythm, movement. It's that springboard that said to me, you've found your place."

5. Pennsylvania Avenue

The percentage of older Americans who vote is higher than any other demographic group. The over-50 crowd is a force to be reckoned with, and women are a significant power bloc. This is an arena where the perspective you gain with age is a great advantage. You know what is important to you and for the world around us. This just might be the perfect time to help clean up the environment; eliminate prejudice; or serve as a guide, a mentor, or an agent of change for younger people. "As my sexual energy has decreased, it's been redirected towards my activism," says Veronica, 70, from

Elmira, New York. "I talk to my Congressional reps on a regular basis. I've been to several peace marches in Washington, D.C. I won't stop until I can't get out of bed."

6. Champs Élysées

Do you dream about whiling away the hours on this famous Paris boulevard over a café au lait? How about floating down the Nile on a barge? Or perhaps the thought of RVing through the national parks is what turns you on. We talked with grandmothers in their 70s who travel with their grandkids and divorcees in their 60s who love cruising with the singles crowd. Travel broadens the mind, enriches the senses, and can be a wonderful way to build your social connections. Charlotte, who is 65, calls Omaha, Nebraska, home, but she has seen the world: "Traveling has supplanted all other pleasures. I have to watch my pennies in order to do so, but I don't mind eating lots of noodles at home if it means I get to take trips."

7. University Plaza

Education influences who we are, what we know, what we believe, how we think, and what we can do. Through learning we find meaning, joy, and connection. Taking or teaching courses at a local college or university, sharing your wisdom with young people, or learning new technological skills is amazingly rewarding. The Internet has unlimited potential as an educational tool. The world of e-mail and chat rooms can allow you to stay linked to old friends and family all over the world and can be an avenue to forming new relationships. "I don't get out as much as I used to, but I spend so much time on-line that I feel really connected to my friends," says Alice, 85, of St. Petersburg, Florida. "I've even participated in an on-line writing group and played bridge on-line. My grandkids think I'm cool."

8. The Garden Path

The little old lady weeding her garden might be a bit of a stereotype, but what about the sturdy, mature woman who oversees the local community vegetable plot or the vibrant senior who runs a commercial wheat farm? Working the soil is a time-honored path to serenity and fulfillment. It is also great exercise and can be another avenue for artistic expression as well as an alternative to spending big bucks in the organic section of your local grocery. "I spend as many hours as I can in the garden. As I've gotten older, I have found the feel of soil between my fingers, the smell of the roses, and even the occasional encounter with an earthworm are all nourishing to my soul," enthuses Judy, 63, of Bainbridge Island, Washington.

9. Freeway to Freedom

While some women are phasing out of their work lives, others are just revving up. They anticipate they will be living well into their 80s, and neither achy joints, nor grandchildren, nor retiring spouses can keep them from pursuing a rewarding vocation. "If you had asked me five years ago what I did, I'd have told you I was a professional community volunteer," says Bertie, 64, of Lexington, Kentucky. "Then, as I was recovering from back surgery and couldn't do much, I began to peruse all my old photos and wondered how the heck I was going to get them organized. I found an organization that helps people keep their mementoes intact. Would you believe I'm now a consultant for that company, and I'm making pretty damn good money at it too?"

10. The United Way

Agencies and faith-based organizations throughout the country bemoan the loss of volunteer labor over the past twenty years. Women who have been focused on their careers and kids and partners had little time to satisfy their generous natures may now have the time to devote to their favorite causes. Claudia, 59, from Colorado Springs, Colorado, felt called to contribute her energy after the recent tsunami. "I just knew I had to do something. That something means I've asked for a leave of absence from my job, and will be spending six months in Southeast Asia building new houses. The only thing that really scares me is the shots I have to take before I leave."

These roads are only a few of the infinite possibilities available for women whose desire has vanished. Take them as suggestions, and tailor them to your own special gifts and energies. Keep your eyes open, and you may well discover uncharted territories that reward your exploration with intriguing adventures.

As you begin any journey, it is always wise to equip yourself with survival skills and a confident attitude. The women who inspired us with their courage and daring; those who found the greatest pleasure in the simple, commonplace acts of living; those who seemed most content as they monitored the shifting tides of their desire were all prepared to redefine sexuality for themselves as they aged.

⌒

From Jay Leno's late-night jokes to Shakespeare's *Hamlet,* diminished desire in the older women is portrayed as one of the humiliating realities of aging. According to Masters and Johnson, AARP polls, physicians, and our own research, a woman's desire most often decreases with age. But as we've just learned, the surprising truth is that for many women, it sure doesn't mean that their sexual self-confidence has disappeared. Women beyond 50 are often confused when their dwindling libidos don't depress them, and they wonder whether they are normal. Because women have been so candid with us, we know that older women who have lost their desire may not have juicy vaginas or perky breasts, but their creativity and their self-assurance do not need to suffer. By bravely exploring new directions, many a mature woman has found new confidence as she continues to blossom.

Sprightly 78-year-old Tina is a political dynamo whose hopes and dreams for her future don't include taking pills or potions for her nonexistent desire. Tina's been widowed for eight years and lives with her son and his family on the East Coast. When we last spoke to her, she was anticipating a trip to her state capitol to advocate for better health care for children. "You can't ever say never, but as far as anticipating an increase in my desire, or even longing for it—no. I don't want to do that at all. I am contented, I am busy and that is good."

Desire Can Surprise You After 50

Who Stays Passionate...And Why

Irma met Harry at the local YMCA. At first they just exchanged glances while pumping iron. Then during a chance encounter at the café, she took his recommendation of the apricot-pineapple-strawberry fruit smoothie with flax seed oil over the nondairy piña colada made with protein powder. A week later they found themselves sitting next to each other at a members' appreciation social. Irma was impressed by Harry's knowledge of the physical effects of aging and even more intrigued by his admission that he was a former workaholic searching for new meaning in his life.

Then, much to her delight, he had asked her out. A date! Sure, it was only for a late afternoon walk and for a drink somewhere afterward, but the idea set her heart racing. She wasn't particularly worried about the tingling sensation she was experiencing; with all of her exercising, she knew her blood pressure was under control. But try as she might, she couldn't remember the last time she'd been so pleasantly perturbed. After all, she was a 70-year-old grandmother of five whose sexual desire had been put to bed when her husband passed away. That was just about the time she had retired. Now she was discovering what many other older women have told us: they've retained the capacity to be turned on to sexual possibilities. The truth is women are never too old to enjoy a happy and healthy sexuality, regardless of their socio-economic status, their age, their marital state, or even their ability to walk without a cane.

Irma was quick to let us know that indeed, her marriage had not been a match made in heaven. Although she'd had a bit of college, she and her husband had married in their early 20s. With a growing family and relatively low-paying jobs, both had been forced to work odd hours to put bread on the table. "We didn't have a lot of time for each other. My husband was my first sexual partner, and I was his first sexual partner. We knew very little, we didn't read about 'it' because you didn't do that. I went for twelve years without having an orgasm. He didn't know how to please me; I didn't know how to tell him, we didn't use the m-word. My grandmother said, 'you just satisfy the man, that is all there is to it,' and I guess I believed her somewhere down deep. My husband and I found out that there was much more to it than that, but it took a long time. We got more relaxed as we got older, so our sex life was better. Maybe the desire I'm now feeling for Harry is something I've hidden away for a long time. I'm really surprised by my newly awakened sexual hunger."

> I have always been very sexually oriented, and as I have gotten older it seems to become more and more prominent.
>
> —*Valerie, 62, lawyer, Atlanta, Georgia*

Joyce is 58 years old. She and Bill moved to Sun City, Arizona, when the last of her five kids got married. "I've only had one sexual partner, and that's my husband of thirty-nine years. So maybe I haven't had the sexual experience that some of my friends have had. But please tell your readers that women 50 and older should not be written off. We are still whole people. We still have desire. My own desire is actually a bit higher than it used to be." Bill and Joyce are both active golfers; in fact, they could be in an ad for living the good life. She is the kind of warm, friendly woman who has maintained lifelong friendships with her high-school buddies. Her marriage has been the exception within her circle, and she has heard many tales from girlfriends who have had unhappy marriages. "Nine times out of ten when a woman over 50 is divorced, she probably has more sexual desire. Maybe her marriage was not such a good one, so she might even have a lot more desire built up in her."

An Unspoken Truth

Women in monogamous relationships (but not married) and those who are dating are more likely than married women to report their sexual desire is greater now than it used to be.

Yes, it's true that most women find that their sexual desire lessens in their post-menopausal years. But this is not a universal truth. Joyce is one of the 14 percent of women of all ages in our study who told us that their sexual desire is greater now than it used to be. In fact, more than half of women in their 50s said that their desire was now either the same or greater than it used to be.

"My sexual desire is so important to my health and well-being. I think it is so primary because I have been sexually active for such a long time and have been with one partner for the last thirty years. It has been a pleasurable and emotionally fulfilling experience. It is very central to my day. I can't remember a time when it was less important, and I can't imagine a time to come when this feeling will change. I had boyfriends pretty early. I didn't have sex when I was a high school freshman, but I was dating by the time I was 13. I had read *Anna Karenina* by the time I was 16. So I knew about great passions." For Kelly, at 51, awareness of sexual desire translates into an enhanced feeling of sexual self-worth.

We met other mature women who, like Kelly, have been able to maintain or reclaim a high level of desire in spite of what our cultural myths, the media, and sometimes even their own partners may be telling them. For many women, the feeling of desire itself is seductive. And they notice that when their desire is high others are drawn to them like moths to a flame. Similar to the mythical Gertrude Stein in Monique Truong's *The Book of Salt,* they begin to carry themselves as though "they are their own object of desire. Such self-induced lust is addictive in its effect..." And the more

The Wet Cigarette

Two old ladies were outside their nursing home having a smoke when it started to rain. One of the ladies pulled out a condom, cut off the end, put it over her cigarette, and continued smoking.

Miriam turned to Agnes and said, "What's that?"

"It's a condom," replied Agnes. This way my cigarette doesn't get wet."

"But where did you get it?" Miriam inquired.

"At the drugstore," said Agnes.

The next day Miriam wheels herself into the local drugstore and announces to the pharmacist that she wants a box of condoms. The guy, obviously embarrassed, looks at her kind of strangely (she is, after all, over 80), but very delicately asks, "What brand do you prefer?"

"Doesn't matter Sonny, as long as it fits a Camel."

passion they exude, the more exhilarated they feel. Raising the level of their sexual energy elevates their sexual self-esteem, which in turn amplifies their desire.

Sophia lives in Indianapolis with her husband of forty-five years and one of her adult children. She told us: "My sexual desire began increasing at 40, and now, 25 years later, it's still sizzling." Her husband's desire has diminished, so she bought the best vibrator on the market, but it still doesn't give her the human touch that she prefers. She loves to flirt with good-looking guys. Luckily, her job provides her with plenty of opportunity to do so. Knowing that men find her attractive is a wonderful boost for her and keeps her feeling vibrant and alive.

Why Do Some Women Have Increased Desire After 50?

June, a 65-year-old divorced waitress with three adult children, learned at a very young age that a man's eyes are the windows to her desire. And men with dark eyes send her soaring. "Black is the color of my desire. It reminds me of the night, and that's when my desire begins to cook."

We asked each of the women who responded to our survey to tell us what factors had had a positive effect on their sexual desire since turning 50. Nearly 50 percent of the women said that no longer worrying about the possibility of getting pregnant had had a positive effect on her desire level. As Maria, a 53-year-old grocery checker, says, "Since I can no longer get pregnant I am more sexually open to trying new kinds of sex." So even though we can feel invisible in this society once we are no longer capable of childbearing, this most concrete of menopausal characteristics can have its benefits.

Women identified a number of lifestyle changes that had led to

Positive Effects on Desire

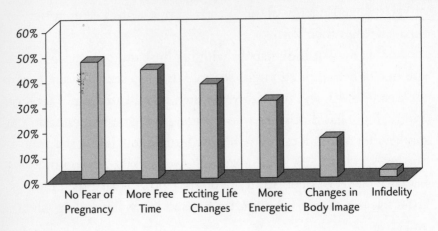

an increase in their desire. The additional free time that came when adult children left home made a positive difference for many women. Some women—about 35 percent of those surveyed—found that they had more energy as they got older and that this had a positive impact. Around 20 percent of our respondents found that positive changes in their body image had caused their sexual desire to blossom. (Negative changes in body image, however, are far more common and powerful—take a look at Chapter 2 for a robust discussion of this topic.)

"If I would have responded to this survey as recently as one year ago, my answers would have been completely different. Shortly before my 55th birthday, my libido changed drastically. I assumed that it was physical but didn't pursue help." We found these comments on the back of a survey submitted by Penny, a 61-year-old bundle of energy who lives in Salt Lake City. She eagerly offered to tell us her story, thinking that her experience might be helpful to other women.

"I'd always greatly enjoyed sex, but it seemed that all desire vanished. Since my husband was slowing down dramatically also, I accepted it. Then, I retired from my high-stress job, got more sleep, and we were presented with an opportunity to live for five months in another country. Miraculously, things turned completely around. Our sex life has been intense and more creative than ever. This did not coincide with my hormone replacement therapy or anything else physical that I can imagine. I would never have believed it." Penny's story is representative of those of a number of women with whom we spoke. Changes in their life circumstances, especially reduction of stress, correlated with increased sexual desire after menopause.

Unspoken Truths

• Women 70 to 79 are significantly more likely than their younger counterparts aged (50 to 69) to explain that not having to worry about getting pregnant anymore has had a positive affect on their sexual desire.

• Women with a household income of under $40,000 are significantly more likely to mention that the inability to get pregnant has had a positive affect on their sexual desire than those with higher incomes.

Who Are the Women Whose Desire Has Increased?

It's no surprise that the women who buck the trend of decreasing desire as they age are an interestingly divergent group. These women's stories are all unique, but the theme of greater desire and, often, more sexual enjoyment in their later years runs through them. We have found that they tend to fall into one of four categories:

1. Women who were surprised by their late-life desire

There are women who have felt a general decline in sexual desire since going through menopause, but who, like Connie, have experienced

Unspoken Truths

• Bisexuals and heterosexuals are more likely than lesbians to anticipate a decrease in their sexual desire in the next ten years.

• The more sexual partners a woman has had in her lifetime, the less likely she is to anticipate a decrease in her sexual desire in the next ten years.

some "sweet surprises" as they have aged. Episodes of heightened desire have overtaken them at unexpected moments: Connie, who is rapidly approaching 60, lives in San Luis Obispo, California, today. This is not where she was raised, however. She describes herself as a "hot-blooded Southerner" who spent most of her first 50 years in Georgia. Connie wrote, "I do not try to understand my increased sexual desire; I do know that I enjoy sexual relations, tenderness, and intimacy with my two partners, much more now than I did ten years ago. But I also feel comfortable masturbating and reaching orgasm with or without them."

Another woman, Barbara, a bubbly 53-year-old empty-nester, told us how she felt after her life changed dramatically because of illness, divorce, and a newfound romance. "I mean, I don't see how women can go without having some kind of sexual contact, whether it is with herself or with somebody else, because it brings a sense of balance and energy. Without orgasm, I can't function; it's like I have to have that release in order to be me." Barbara experienced menopause in her thirties after undergoing chemotherapy, but she didn't see any lessening in her libido as a result." I think there has to be that connection with the right person to trigger it. But women can look for that. If anybody had told me that I would feel what I feel now when I was younger, I would have said, 'You're crazy!'

"I remember when I visited my sister-in-law a number of years ago, and she was just recently divorced and she said it was just horrible. She had so much sexual energy, and there was nowhere for it to go! And I was still married at the time so I didn't know what she was talking about. When I got divorced, I found out! I don't think I had as much sexual desire with my husband as I do with my current partner, Rick. But there is an age difference. For me there was a 12-year gap of no sex, having desire but not having it fulfilled.

"I can't even think of what would turn off my desire since I am enjoying life—and sex—so much now."

2. Women who have always had a high level of desire

There are women whose level of desire has been high all their lives and has remained so as they have aged, even if the intensity of their sexual response has diminished.

"There is a tremendous difference between a 50-year-old and an 80-year-old woman. The desire for me has always remained. But the intensity has waned," remarked Ada, a New Yorker who mourns her youthful lustiness. She pines for the days when her sexual response was at a fever pitch. "You know, it used to be that the force of my orgasm could literally bring me to tears."

Sixty-two-year-old Olive hails from Wyoming. Her story of her infidelity and its effect on her desire and her self-worth is revealing. "I have always been very sexually oriented, and as I have gotten older it seems to become more prominent. I have more urges, more often I feel like I want to have sex a lot. I was always boy crazy from about the age of ten on up. I wanted to run with

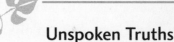

Unspoken Truths

• A woman's relationship status does not deter her from wishing she had sex with a partner more often.

• Geographic location and sexual preference do not have an effect on how often a woman would like to have sex with her partner.

the boys. I wanted to play baseball. I wanted to be where they were. I always had lots of boyfriends. I always was where the action was.

"I was taught to suppress my sexual desire as a teenager. I was president of my Methodist Youth Fellowship group, and I was very active in the church. I believed that it was a sin to have sex before you married. I did have it once, maybe a couple of times, but nothing much because I did see it as something that was so wrong. My religious background—more than my parent's teachings—really kept me from having sex, I guess.

"When I married my husband I was 19 and he was 17. We were really young, terribly, terribly inexperienced, and just thought we had to get married to have sex. And we did get married. Neither of us really knew what we were doing sexually. Back in those days there wasn't much available to help. There wasn't much written, so you only learned from what you heard through a few girlfriends talking. Then, after I got older, I found and read some materials that I had never been privy to before. Boy was I curious.

"Then, after I turned 40, I met someone who enlightened me a lot. I met a man—David—who wasn't afraid to try things because he had been around a lot. He introduced me to many things that were very enjoyable. I had no idea that I could have an orgasm until I was 40. He made me believe in myself. I liked his openness and his willingness to share his knowledge... and of course my desire is higher, probably because of what he's taught me... But he is a scoundrel! I did go home and I taught my husband about it. But I didn't tell him I learned it from another man."

Fifty-seven-year-old LuAnn's tale is sadly one we heard many times. "I feel cheated because I am a very sexual person and my husband cannot, so I am starved for sex. I have been with a lover a couple of times in the past a year but then guilt takes over. I just feel cheated."

3. Women who have plenty of desire ... but no partner to share it with

There are women whose desire has increased but who are not in a sexual relationship where they can act on it.

Bobbie, a 58-year-old divorced tax accountant with three young grandchildren, says, "Well, it is very high, but when I can't do so much about it I cool off. At my age, I believe it is important to have a well-rounded, healthy sexuality. I am a very, very monogamous person. I have had very few sexual partners—just my husbands. I wouldn't have risked my marriages for being in bed with someone else. So now I simply turn myself off."

There can be real disadvantages for a sexually energized woman who is on her own. Caroline, a 55-year-old software programmer, had been looking forward to the fabled decline in desire she expected after menopause, but for her it didn't happen. "I get angry sometimes because my sexual desire is so high. I think there should be a pill the opposite of Viagra for people like me. According to the media, it's the man who has to have it all the time. They don't talk about the woman who is highly sexed."

4. Women who find a new relationship—and renewed desire—after 50

There are women who thought their sexual desire was long gone but found that with a new relationship, desire resurfaced with surprising intensity:

Marion, who had been single for 20 years after divorcing her husband, had come to believe that her sexual life was over. She had plenty of women friends and male companions, but sex was not even an option she considered. It wasn't that she missed it; it was more like it just didn't exist. Then at her grandson's wedding, she discovered that Harold, the fellow whom she had dated for a short

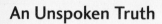

An Unspoken Truth

Women who are monogamous, are dating, have multiple partners, or are separated are significantly more likely than those who are married to indicate there has been a slight to moderate increase in their satisfaction with sex after reaching 50 years of age.

time before the war disrupted their lives, had been widowed himself. The old romantic feelings resurfaced with shocking speed. Now 80, Marion told us: "Our first kiss was electrifying, and it's been that way ever since."

When we looked closely at the survey responses from women aged 80 to 95, we found that more of the women in this age group stated that their desire was greater than it used to be than did women in their 50s, 60s, or 70s. This data is reinforced by many stories we heard from octogenarians who described resurgence in their sexual desire after decades of decline.

Could This Be You?

Okay, so what's going on here? Do women like Irma and Marion have a different hormonal makeup from the majority of older women? Or can we all expect to reignite our sexual flames in our golden years? When asked to think back over their level of sexual desire during the past decade, most women could identify a general decline that included many points when their desire peaked. But the causes for this diminishment in desire and accompanying peaks and valleys are elusive. Researchers aim to demonstrate there is often a hormonal cause. A 1998 study conducted by M. R. Jiroutek and his colleagues measured changes in reproductive hormones and SHBG (sex-hormone binding globulin) in a group of women who had gone through natural menopause. The researchers followed these women over a ten-year period and found that "the trend in hormone concentrations shows no set pattern with aging in the postmenopausal years." In fact, according to his study, testosterone levels of women might even show a slight increase. A more recent study, conducted by Susan Davis et al. and reported in the *Journal of the American Medical Association* on July 6, 2005, was designed to determine whether women with self-reported low sexual desire have lower levels of androgen (a sex hormone) than other women. They found no evidence of association between low levels of serum and free testosterone and low levels of sexual desire or satisfaction.

It's becoming clearer that hormonal swings and testosterone levels do not account for the whole story. We know that women's sexual desire cannot be reduced to a solely chemical explanation. In fact, lots of women told us that they continued to feel sexual desire, but they faced many barriers that were so formidable that they no longer enjoyed sex.

For some, the problem is incontinence. The pelvic floor muscles provide support for the vagina, urethra, uterus, and bowel—and help keep them in their correct position. As we age, all our muscles tend to lose tone and strength if we don't exercise them specifically. The effect of weakened pelvic floor muscles can be quite devastating as bladder and bowel leakage, and decreased sexual sensation often occur when they loosen. Incontinence is a condition that most women are reluctant to talk

Incontinence

If you're plagued with this infirmity, we encourage you to talk to both your partner and your doctor about what's been happening to you. There are a number of things your physician might suggest. Some are simple: urinating before you have sex, doing Kegel exercises regularly, and changing your position. Other treatment options include getting help from a specially trained physical therapist, biofeedback, medications, and surgery.

about with their friends, their partners, or their doctors, but leakage is a pretty common experience, especially for women over 50. Can it affect a woman's desire? According to *The Incontinence Solution: Answers for Women of All Ages* by Parker, Rosenman, and Parker, "one study found that almost 70 percent of women with urgency or urge incontinence (the result of an overactive bladder) had unsatisfying sexual relations; 20 percent of women with stress incontinence had this complaint." One woman told us, "I felt so embarrassed that I might dribble a bit when I had an orgasm, so I started to avoid having sex. I really didn't feel very clean—or very desirable. I finally had the guts to talk to my husband; luckily he was pretty understanding."

For a somewhat smaller percentage, sexual intercourse is actually painful. As we explained in Chapter 2, women's physiology changes fairly markedly with the onset of menopause. A decrease in the amount of estrogen a woman produces may reduce genital sensations, a dry vagina can become irritated by penetration, and thinning of the vaginal walls may cause bleeding. A women's desire may be high, but the sex act itself can be excruciating. Who wants to engage in something that is going to lead to soreness? After a while, many a woman simply puts her desire on the back shelf. She may dust it off every now and again, but over time, she may even forget where she's put it.

Some women still long to have sex with their partner but recognize they and their partners are mismatched when it comes to desire levels. One may be in the mood, but not necessarily when the other one is. For example, Karen, a 54-year-old divorced mother of four, runs an antique shop in upstate New York. She admits that she's had a fair number of partners, "Somewhere in the neighborhood of twenty or twenty-five, I think." When she was younger, Karen struggled with her level of desire; now that she is older, she's grown more comfortable and accepting. "I think I am now much more open and relaxed about sex and the taboos that were laid heavily on me as a young person I have discarded. I have been more able to express myself sexually with my partner. I had this one guy who I was dating after my divorce. I enjoyed having sex with him quite a bit and he was very generous, and I always had an orgasm and I loved having sex with him. Somewhere in the relationship it seemed like his desire dropped off. And then, when I tried to initiate it sometimes he would respond and then he would get annoyed and said I wanted sex too much. And then it made me feel like I couldn't initiate it. And what seemed comfortable for him in terms of the frequency to me was far too little, and I decided that I wasn't over-sexed, but that he was undersexed... we just weren't right for each other."

Even in the face of the numerous challenges that come with aging and can interfere with sexual feelings, many of us yearn to reignite our passionate lives. Given the choice, many women would rather be like Joyce and feel that old zing than to accept that our sexual energy is on the wane. Is there anything to be done? Do we still have the ability to flip the switch to the on position, even for a while? It may not be as easy or instantaneous as turning on a light, but you can manipulate your environment and your attitude so that getting turned on yourself becomes much more likely.

Keeping the Lust Alive

In our study, women from 50 to 95—yes, even women 80 years of age and older—indicated that they were interested in increasing the number of times they have sex with a partner. On average women over 50 years of age reported they had sex 50 times over the past year (approximately once a week); however, they would like to be having sex 88 times a year (nearly twice a week). And the octogenarians wanted to increase their sexual encounters from nearly once a month to more often than once a week.

We pass on these tales of women like Irma and Marion because they can serve as role models. The attitudes these lusty older women hold and the approaches they have taken to maintain and reawaken their sexual fervor are instructive and encouraging. If you long to feel greater sexual drive or wish to maintain the level of desire you have today, consider these guidelines:

1. **Pay close attention to your sexual sensations.** "Attention is the ultimate aphrodisiac," advises Marge, 63. She was talking about the power of male attention, but her comment applies more broadly. We can choose to ignore the mild signals of arousal our bodies send, or we can fan the sparks into flames. Sexual sensation is the ultimate combo of the mental and the physical. Sexual thoughts and fantasies can be powerful stimulators. It can take practice, but what have you got to lose?

Rather than following the usual prescriptions for stimulating romance—candlelight dinners or taking a warm bath together (not be scoffed at, of course), Lori, a 53-year-old whose head is framed by a tangle of salt-and-pepper curls, says she and her husband began to pay attention to small things that turned them on. "Country music had always turned me on, and to this day it still does...My husband and I went to a dance to celebrate my 50th birthday a few years ago. A live band was playing. The vocalist was singing 'Can I Have This Dance for the Rest of My Life?' I almost swooned. Now, if we want to get in the mood, we definitely turn on the country music. And we're already planning the songs we want to dance to when I celebrate my 55th."

2. **Find new ways to savor your sensuality.** You probably have had your fair share of ups and downs, both in life and in sexual desire. Sometime in the past you may have felt like an asexual being; sometimes you may have felt the fullness of your sexuality blossom when you started a new relationship. You're now at a point in your

life when your sexuality may take a different form of expression than it did in your youth. After all, we can get turned on pretty fast when we're in our 20s, but in later life, we move at a gentler pace. At 60 or 70, after years of sexual experience, we can express our sexuality in a more advanced, more refined mode.

Gloria, named after her conservative grandmother who taught her that sex was only for procreation and not enjoyment, has broken the spell of the past. At 60, she feels she is just coming into her own. She told us, "What turns me on? Oh, sometimes a glance, a fleeting look, many times just a touch, will get me going. Even a glimpse of an attractive man across the room can set a spark off. Not that I would act on it— my second husband and I really have a great thing going—but I love that flicker of excitement and energy! My family was conservative, very religiously conservative. It was rural Baptist. No movies, no smoking, no dancing…we played cards, but you weren't supposed to. Then it dawned on me, 'wait a minute, that is my parents' philosophy and my parents' religion. The decisions have to be mine.' And I try to live that to this day."

> When it comes to sex and older women, a lot of what I read is hogwash…Although I've been widowed for years, I still get turned on when I see a man in a blue shirt…and he responds to my glance.
>
> —*Consuelo, 74,*
> *San Pedro, California*

Some women have acknowledged that their sexual cravings were pretty high from an early age and thought they would sail through the rest of their lives in much the same mode. Now, however, they are facing some new challenges. Jodenne is a never-been-married social service agency executive from Sacramento, California, facing some newfound dilemmas. Flamboyant and festive in a hot pink suit, she says, "I think other women are more triggered by the heart, and the need for security and status. I feel very, very secure

> In my 20s I was only attracted to men who were not physically threatening to me, who could not hurt me. I have never been hurt, physically by a man...never been hit, never been bullied around in a way that felt threatening. And yet now I find myself more turned on to men who are better built. And I don't know what that's about. Although I used to be very thin myself and I am not so much anymore. I am more normal weight so maybe that is all this is. I feel stronger. I could resist.
>
> —*Adrianne, 59, Washington, D.C.*

and I don't need men. I am very independent of men economically. I don't need a man's power to be powerful, yet I find power to be a tremendous aphrodisiac.

"I have always taken sex for granted. I'm a sexual person, always wanting to be having sex and never really saw myself with one person for the rest of my life. Now I'm not so sure. I feel more settled down and less in need of having a variety of experiences."

3. **Know that you can recover from grief.** Bouncing back sexually after divorce or the death of a partner or spouse is not easy. It tests the strength and resilience of even the hardiest of souls. Yet many women are exhilarated to find that after a period of grieving, their sexual desire is in full swing, and their self-esteem is lifted to new heights. Adele, 69, was delighted and a bit startled by the positive effect of her new marriage. "I remarried more than two years ago and experienced increased sexual desire. My previous husband (now deceased) was impotent and in poor health during the last decade of our marriage. I am currently married to a wonderful man who fulfills me in all ways, sexual and non-sexual. I am extremely fortunate to have such a wonderful husband at this stage of my life."

Another woman, Vi, is 52 and also marveling at her good fortune. "After my divorce I believed I would never have sex again and it really concerned me a lot. Of course, since it didn't work out that way, I am really happy about that. I plan to be having and enjoying sex for as long as I'm able—until 100 if possible."

4. **Take time to savor memorable moments, both sexual and nonsexual.** Is it really any surprise that the personals ads that clog the newspapers and websites are full of older men and women who describe themselves as loving long walks on the beach or strolling through antique shops? To some extent, the phrases have become code words whose meaning isn't lost on the reader. They are well aware that a seaside amble may very well mean "I'd like to have sex with you." But because the most lasting sexual intimacy builds from shared joys, savoring time together can be the ultimate form of foreplay.

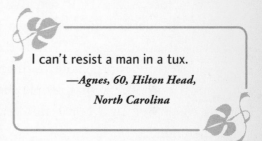

I can't resist a man in a tux.
—*Agnes, 60, Hilton Head, North Carolina*

Talking about memorable sexual moments can have a stimulating effect on your desire. You may wish to try asking your spouse or partner, "Since we've been together, what is your favorite story about your own desire?" or "Which of our sexual escapades is your favorite?" Recalling experiences of mutual sexual passion can be your private channel for reigniting your romance.

As 59-year-old Iris and her husband discovered, even stealing a few minutes from a busy day can be a powerful love potion. "It used to be that obligations would overwhelm us. I figured out that I felt pretty sexual about three times a week, but we'd generally act on that desire only about once a week. We had all these obligations that came before our pleasure and intimacy. It was so sad—so we figured out that when we felt the desire, we would just stop what we were doing for five minutes. Now we give each other a hug, and sometimes a deep passionate kiss. We make plans to act on our feelings later; then we just go back to attending to our obligations. Now I no longer feel sad or think that I've been cheated out of an orgasm. We've got promises to keep before we sleep."

⌒⟶

Sexual adventures and longing are not confined to women with buff, wrinkleless, young bodies. Many mature women are ecstatic to find that they are experiencing heightened desire, increased self-confidence, and soaring sexual satisfaction beyond 50. Betsy, a 54-year-old married mother of two adult children, is a dog groomer from Bend, Oregon. "There is this myth that when you get older your sexual desire goes down dramatically. I don't think that is true, and I don't think that people should believe that. It may happen to some women...but I think it is probably more idiosyncratic than not."

Some of the women we talked to at house gatherings and interviewed in depth suggested that certain aftershaves, the husky voice of an actor, or the rustle of a fabric similar to a long-forgotten party dress could trigger flames of desire that could grow into a raging inferno. Some were on hormones or took testosterone and attributed their renewed interest to their "magic pills." But many were not taking such medications. Some were divorced and had rediscovered lost passion with a new romance. "I would say that my increase in desire and satisfaction is less a function of age than leaving a marriage in which I was very unhappy and unsatisfied and enjoying a wonderful sexual relationship with my new husband for the past nine years," said Sherry, a 62-year-old clerk from Tucson.

Others have kept the flame alive during the course of very long-term, monogamous relationships. Margaret, a retired teacher from Grand Haven, Michigan, told us, "I have always had high libido. I've loved making love with my husband of 42 years and still do."

For some women, desire that had been at low ebb suddenly surged with the coming of menopause. Others continue to count themselves among the lucky ones whose desire has always been at a fever pitch. The women who expressed positive expectations about what will happen to their sexual desire over the next ten years are anticipating a sexually fulfilling future. Most of these women are radiating an aura of sexiness despite gnarly fingers, thinning hair, flabby thighs, medicine cabinets full of pills, and admonishments from their children to act their age. Filled with a sense of awe and wonder, they may be a bit slower, a bit more stooped, but their prospects are good and their options unlimited.

Truth #5

Masturbation Can Keep You Independent

Who Are the Over-50 Self-Pleasuring Queens?

In the early days of our research project, we received an intriguing message on our voicemail: "I'd like to participate in your study. I think it's important for other women to know about my experience. I've never told another soul on the planet about this." When we returned the call, we learned that Sally, the 56-year-old owner of an accounting firm, wanted to talk to us about masturbation.

"When my daughter went off to college, I bought a vibrator. I never...I'm not a wild and crazy woman. I've been totally monogamous all my life. I've never done anything too strange or different in this way. And I loved it so much...It was much better than anything I experienced with my husband. I want to tell other women about it." Married to Ted for twenty-seven years, Sally was sure that her limited exposure to self-pleasuring was typical of many women her age.

Sally had received one of our surveys in the mail and recognized an opportunity to share her private discovery. Her earnest and sincere wish was to tell other older women about the benefits of using a vibrator. A well-educated, sophisticated woman who had challenged many stereotypes as the owner of a typically male-dominated business, Sally had not fully appreciated her own sexual responsiveness until she learned about masturbation. Like many other women, she didn't gain this knowledge until she was well into menopause.

"Although I haven't had experiences with other men, I feel that my husband has never been much of a lover. He's not very communicative, and he's pretty much focused on his own pleasure. Over the years we've been very busy people, involved in various professional things, raising the kids, and living our life. So sex had become less and less important and rather perfunctory. I started thinking about the fact that I never felt that I really had these orgasms, you know, that everyone talks about. And I got curious I guess. I found a percent off coupon in the newspaper, believe it or not, for a sex toy shop...and that's how it all started."

"Now I feel I can take care of my sexual comforts and pleasures by myself far better than I ever could with my husband. As I've gotten older, I don't feel like I want to use the vibrator or have sex real often. I'm not that into it; I have a busy, active, interesting life and I don't dwell on it or think about it particularly. I use it once every one or two weeks depending on when I have private time. My husband doesn't know about it. He's not doing real well sexually himself, he's had trouble maintaining an erection as he's gotten older, so he's not real interested in sex either. Our relationship is OK. I'm sure we'll be rocking on the porch together in our old age."

The role masturbation plays in the lives of women over 50 runs the gamut. For many women, giving themselves sexual pleasure has become increasingly important as they have aged—they've overcome old taboos and are on a mission to let other women know about such joys. Some find masturbation is as pleasurable as it has always been, but they just don't do it as often. For others, masturbation is unrewarding, unappealing, or simply not acceptable to them.

Regardless of their own experience with masturbation, few women over 50 realize how much of a role it plays in the sexual lives of their peers.

Attitudes, Platitudes, and Taboos

Sally's story about her masturbation discovery reflects the impact societal taboos have had on many older women. It's not as though TV sitcoms, thousands of websites, the tabloids, and even some magazines totally avoid the topic—but there's a "wink-wink" aspect to it, reserving the practice for the young and hormonally overwhelmed.

> Somewhere along the way I got a negative message. I've tried but it never really seemed to work.
> I would think to myself, if my husband does this to me and he does such a great job, why can't I do the great job? But it just doesn't work.
>
> —*Bonnie, 64, raised a Catholic, converted to Judaism*

The political climate in the United States isn't conducive to introducing masturbation as an aspect of sexual education, either. It wasn't that long ago (December 1994) that the brief tenure of former U.S. surgeon general Jocelyn Elders came to an abrupt end. Her statement "masturbation is part of human sexuality and a part of something that perhaps should be taught" got her in the political dog house, prompting former president Bill Clinton to ask for her resignation. No other surgeon general or politician at the national level has dared utter a word about it in a public setting since.

The degree of comfort older women feel with masturbation is frequently influenced by powerful religious beliefs and cultural myths that generally relegate it to the pile of unmentionables. We heard stories from women whose upbringing led them to feel tremendous shame and guilt because of the pleasure they felt when masturbating. For example, Janis, a 55-year-old bisexual woman raised in Denver, told us about the repercussions of her upbringing: "I was raised to believe that masturbation was a mortal sin. I refrained from touching myself all through my teens and early twenties. My first sexual experiences were not very positive and I really thought there was something wrong with me. It took me a long time to understand that I was OK; I just didn't know how my own body worked. Now, being able to masturbate without guilt and to know that it's good for all of my being has kept my sexual desire awake. It makes me know that that piece of myself is still alive, and it's also an incredible tension release."

Also in her 50s, Malka grew up in a very different cultural milieu, yet she got a lot of negative messages about self-pleasuring as well. Hers was an Orthodox Jewish household in Queens, New York. She told us, "It had such a bad rap when I was growing up. [But] people masturbate because they don't have a partner, or because they're unsatisfied with the one they do have, not because they're bad. Sometimes, nobody knows what I want as much as I do."

> Masturbation for me has been a wonderful gift.
> —*Madelyn, 62, Erie, Pennsylvania*

A very different perspective on the role of religious teaching about sexuality and masturbation was articulated by 52-year-old Kathleen, who was raised as a member of the Church of Jesus Christ of Latter-Day Saints. Now living in Idaho, she said, "I was a very early masturbator; I started when I was a little girl. And I continued to masturbate throughout my first marriage. But before I met my second husband I made a conscious effort to control that and not do it. It was part of my coming back into my religious faith. I began to learn to master that. It was a total self-control thing for me.

I kind of likened it to a factory that I just sort of shut down. I just taught myself not to do that, not to stimulate myself that way. And that was a big thing for me to overcome.

"But I will tell you what; it made it very much easier for my husband and me not to have sexual relations before we were married. I think that really helped me because it was really hard for us to wait until we were married, but we did. This is very unusual for a lot of people, I know, especially when you have been married before like we had. But it was a commitment that I had made to myself and to God. I wanted to do it right this time and I felt like a virgin on our wedding night. It was the oddest thing. I know it sounds really strange. But I really did and it was really cool."

Away Too Much

Tired of a listless sex life, the man came right out and asked his wife during a recent lovemaking session, "How come you never tell me when you have an orgasm?" She glanced at him casually and replied, "You're never home!"

Forty years ago the United States Supreme Court ruled that *Fanny Hill*, a book originally published in 1749, was not pornographic even though it contained, among other sexually explicit scenes, some pretty graphic descriptions of female masturbation. But court rulings do not prevent us from absorbing negative messages. Old teachings and attitudes about this subject are powerfully inhibiting as one African-American woman, a 54-year-old widow, said: "I'll try it occasionally and it's fulfilling for me. Ten years ago I probably wouldn't have told you that. I wouldn't have been open; its something I wouldn't have talked about—growing up in a culture where it's something of a taboo, you know old wives tales about going crazy and all that. In the South (I grew up in Tennessee), in the context of the church, there was no such thing as sexual feelings and certainly not masturbation—you never talked about it."

Cultural stereotyping prevented Donna from appreciating the benefits of masturbation until later in life. "I would say that is something that I discovered relatively late. Not until I was in my 40s did I start masturbating with any frequency. I don't know why exactly except in the culture I grew up in masturbation was considered masculine. It just never occurred to me. But I had been sexually active since I was 19. And so, I guess I felt that my needs were pretty much met. Then I hit my 40s and I had this surge of sexual energy. I don't know where it came from, but it was there. I knew of course that my husband—over the years, I'm sure he was masturbating, and that didn't particularly bother me. I had this surge of energy myself so I started doing it too, and it became pretty important to me."

With words like *sin* and *taboo* so strongly attached to masturbation, it's not surprising that women tend to keep this topic pretty hushed up. Yet as with so many subjects that were once considered improper in polite conversation, speaking openly about self-pleasuring can be beneficial in many ways.

The Benefits of Being "A Woman of Independent Means"

There may not be any causal link between masturbation and long life, but then again, who knows? Almost all of the women over age 80 we interviewed acknowledged that masturbation has played an important role in their lives!

As our bodies go through the multiple changes that characterize the post-menopausal years, the substantial differences in sexual responsiveness and levels of desire can be disheartening and sometimes even frightening to women. If we're not comfortable with our body image, if we're coping with physical illness and disability, or if we don't understand how physiological aging affects our sexual sensations, it's easy to reach the conclusion that our sex lives are over when the same old patterns of stimulation no longer lead to the same level of excitement or satisfaction. While you may find it helpful to learn that most older women experience these changes, the specifics of how your particular body is aging sexually are best uncovered on your own. This is the educational value of masturbation. Exploring how to pleasure yourself sexually in the new terrain of the beyond-50 years provides you with direct feedback that instructs and informs. Whether you chose to use this information to enlighten your partner about how to please you, or to enhance your own private delights, self-pleasuring can provide personal evidence that your sexual responsiveness may be altered, but it is still alive.

Doris is a 63-year-old mother of three and grandmother of two who lives with her husband in the starkly beautiful country around Flagstaff, Arizona. She is a hardworking outdoorswoman who spends the better part of her days with her horses. "I started masturbating—I think it would be considered late for some people—probably not until my early 20s. It's always been part of who I am, even when I've had a sexual partner, the same way that I felt if they wanted to, that was part of their sexuality. It didn't diminish what we had together. As I've gotten older, as with all aspects of my sexuality, it's diminished. I've required more stimulation; I need a vibrator now, when I was younger I didn't. It's still part of my repertoire of expression, and along with all of my expression, it's decreased."

Is there an age when most women discover the delights of self-pleasuring? Probably not, but we often heard from women we interviewed that they believed they had discovered self-pleasuring much later than most. They said, "I was kind of old" or "I was a late bloomer" when they were talking about masturbation. We reassured these women that it's never too late to learn, because we had already talked to Evie. At 92, she was bright and eager and had anticipated our conversation at her San Diego cottage with great excitement. With a giggle, she said, "Oh, I'm just so pleased that you've come. I love the idea of telling you my story." She was nearly 80 years old before she discovered self-pleasuring. Evie revealed that she was also an author, and after we had gotten to know one another a bit, she offered to write the rest of the story. Her own words tell it best:

"To me, menopause didn't affect my sex life one way or the other, but somewhere in our sixties or early seventies, sex tapered off. Fred lost interest. I read an article in a women's magazine on how to rekindle the fire. So, one day when he came home from work I met him at the door wearing nothing but Saran Wrap. He said, 'Won't you catch cold?' and headed for the liquor cabinet.

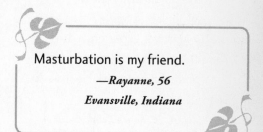

Masturbation is my friend.
—*Rayanne, 56*
Evansville, Indiana

"Eventually, I confided in my friend Lil, 'I still have urges. Don't you? What's to be done about it?'

"'Unless we find Latin lovers, there's only one way out.'

"'What's that?'

"She hesitated, and then whispered, 'Masturbate.'

"I was shocked. 'Do you?'

"Although we had been best friends for forty years, she blushed and nodded.

"The first time I tried, I felt embarrassed, guilty. When I was a kid it was something bad. Boys were told that they'd go blind and nice girls never touched 'those parts' except to wash.

"But Mother Nature's urges were strong. Evenings, after Fred retired, I'd put a Dean Martin or Frank Sinatra record on the stereo, pour a glass of wine, and light a candle. Gradually self-gratification became easier.

"At my eightieth birthday Lil said, 'You're doing it, aren't you?'

"'What?' I asked, feigning wide-eyed innocence.

"She laughed. 'I can tell. You're more relaxed. You go around with a *Mona Lisa* smile on your face.'"

"When I was almost 90, I read a book about self-pleasuring by Dr. Ruth Westheimer and bought her vibrator kit. This added new highs, and the first time I tried it I was so carried away I was afraid I'd have a heart attack. I thought, *how embarrassing to be found dead in bed with the vibrator humming. Then again, what a way to go!*"

In a later phone conversation with Evie, who we've come to think of as our "masturbation queen," she mused, "You know, I don't understand why we don't talk about this more. They talk about such awful things on television and in the movies, about sadomasochism and rape, but this is just nice. No one gets hurt; it's only for yourself."

> I had been single for a couple of years and one day I just tried it. After I practiced a little bit I was able to stimulate myself to orgasm, which at age 47 was a pretty amazing experience. It is something that I still enjoy with my wonderful husband. He likes to share it with me.
>
> —*Naomi, 55, South Bend, Indiana*

Evie envisioned helping us start a masturbation movement, so to speak, that would reach the dreary halls of assisted-living homes for the elderly across the country. "All those sad, old souls who spend their days sitting in chairs with blankets on their laps. Think of it—they could be enjoying themselves and no one would be the wiser. Why not?"

The Art of Talking About It

In her 1976 book *The Hite Report*, Shere Hite wrote: "We have arrived at a point where it has become acceptable for women to enjoy sex, as long as we are fulfilling our roles as women—that is, giving pleasure to men, participating in mutual activities. Perhaps in the future we will be able to feel we have the right to enjoy masturbation too." It's been 30 years since Hite made this hesitant projection for women's increased ownership of their sexual lives. Has her version of the future finally arrived?

The answer is both yes and no. We asked women, "What role has masturbation played in your life?" Sixty-nine percent of the replies to this question were like Jane's: "a huge role." Many told us this aspect of their sexual repertoire has been essential to maintaining healthy self-esteem at times when they were without a mate. For others, it was just a routine part of their sexual lives whether they were partnered or not. And yet, most women openly acknowledged that they had never talked about this with anyone until our conversation. What does this say about our sense that we have "the right to enjoy masturbation"? When asked directly we may admit to it, yet there is still some sense of mortification because we've been "caught" with our hands in our pants.

A number of older women acknowledged that they find it hard to even say the word *masturbation* aloud. They may never have used it in a sentence, especially in a sentence that also contained the word *I*. Referring to it as "the m word" or "self-pleasuring" made it a more acceptable. Virginia, an 85-year-old Ivy League graduate with 60 years of professional work behind her,

> When I learned about my own thing, about masturbation, I was like, oooooh…I learned through experimentation. Actually I was with a gentleman. He went to answer the phone and there I was waiting and waiting. I thought, you know what, 'I'm not going to wait here forever,' so I just started to experiment with myself, explore and 'Voilà!' I found the magic button. When he came back, I said, 'you know what, I'm leaving—you were on the phone forever!'
>
> —*Angela, 64, Eureka, California*

wrote: "When my sexual desire is high, I'll either ignore it or 'pleasure myself.' The technical name for this has such an unpleasant sound, no wonder people shy away from pronouncing it."

Openly talking about masturbation with a sexual partner or with other female friends can require significant fortitude and willingness to challenge a major societal taboo. Letting your sexual partner in on the secrets about your body's responsiveness that you have learned through masturbation can be tricky. How will he take it if you tell him that you need a different kind of touch than what he has been using for years? Will it upset your relationship to know that now that you are older, your body may not respond to intercourse with the same pleasure as it does to the use of a vibrator? If you have a male partner who is over 50 himself, remember that his body is changing also. His responsiveness to your touch is different from what it was as a younger man. This may be a difficult conversation to initiate, but it can lead to both of you feeling more comfortable and less pressured. (See Chapter 8 for more about initiating conversations with your partner.)

"In my marriage I would masturbate secretly because I didn't want my husband to know I was doing it. I felt he would be angry with me and feel I was robbing him of something. I felt very ambivalent." Stella told her story with great enthusiasm, eager to inform other women that even at 82 they can experience passionate sexual feelings. She offered herself as an example. "I've learned a totally different attitude with my lover. He masturbates on occasion, perfectly comfortably, and I do too and he loves it. It's a turn-on for him. So, it works out very well. I got that comfort from him; it was contagious. He made it easy for me to talk about."

The condemnation heaped on self-pleasuring can rob it of its potential as a source of self-knowledge and enhanced sexual self-esteem. But as we've heard, older women are coming to appreciate its benefits. We have met many women who, as they have aged, have delighted in a burgeoning brazenness that has allowed them to overcome such embarrassment and to storm the walls of convention.

Stayin' Alive?

Several of the women we talked to about masturbation were widows at the time of our conversations with them. Most had married young; some had had fulfilling sexual lives with their husbands; others had not. Self-pleasuring was described by most of them as a way to stay connected to their sexual selves regardless of how active or satisfying their partnered sex was.

Eleanor runs a charming bed and breakfast near the campus of a small college in a rather isolated Midwestern town. She's lived in the area for all of her 73 years and has survived two husbands and raised four children in the rambling farmhouse that is now her main source of income. A small, spry woman with sparkling brown eyes, Eleanor looks closer to 60 than 70. As we talked over coffee one morning, she told this tale about her and her 87-year-old friend, Sadie: "Just the other day, I'd been reading a Nora Roberts novel and I felt 'it'—you know, that sexual tingle—and I thought 'I'm not dead!' I said to Sadie, 'That Nora Roberts, she's something!' And Sadie nodded. Later on, Sadie was napping in her chair, and when she woke up I said, 'You must have been having a good dream, because you had a smile on your face.' And she said, 'I was being seduced! It's so nice to be

An Unspoken Truth

Women who tend to have fewer sexual thoughts or fantasies are: married, have had fewer sexual partners, have stopped taking HRT.

able to feel that all by yourself even at my age.' It's like that with self-pleasuring—you just need to feel that once in a while and you know you're still alive."

Like Sadie, women talked to us about having sexual fantasies and dreams throughout the last five decades of life. The majority (55 percent) of women we surveyed have sexual thoughts or fantasies at least once a week; 11 percent have fantasies daily.

For some women, self-pleasuring is an unconscious, uniquely pleasurably act that occurs during sleep. *The Kinsey Institute New Report on Sex* by June M. Reinisch, Ph.D., states: "It is estimated that about 40 percent of women have had orgasms during sleep, and they seem to become more common as a woman gets older." Megan, an 84-year-old divorcee from Waco, Texas, told us, "Masturbation hasn't played much of a role in my sexual desire. I have gone through two or three periods in my life over the last fifty years when I did more experimentation with that, but it felt kind of clumsy and was never a very fulfilling thing, so I pretty much don't do it. However I do have sexual dreams. They generally involve somebody I have known in the past, and in the dream itself I am having sex with the person...and then I will wake up because I have had an orgasm. It is pretty much just a mental thing. I think that it happens not as frequently as it used to. I would say it probably has been a couple of months since the last time I had that. I don't really see that as physical masturbation, but it does happen."

Among the benefits of masturbation is the maintenance of vaginal health. As Dr. Christiane Northrup says in her book *The Wisdom of Menopause,* "Women who masturbate in ways that involve vaginal penetration often maintain excellent vaginal function even when not in a relationship that involves sexual intercourse." Self-pleasuring can also provide a form of physical therapy. Frequently women said their sexual sensations had been deadened by illness or by chemotherapy. For many, masturbation was essential to their healing.

At one of our house gatherings, Gretchen described how

wonderfully rejuvenating it was for her to get reacquainted with her body as a source of sexual pleasure. The group listened intently as she spoke. "I'd been in a virtually sexless marriage for over 20 years," she said. Diagnosed with uterine cancer shortly after she divorced her husband, she had surgery and chemotherapy, which left her vagina desiccated and very tender. When she was finally finished with all the treatment, she met "the love of my life"—a kind and patient man. She wanted to be sexual with him. But it just didn't work.

"My doctor is an angel from heaven," she told the group. "He told me, 'Get yourself a vibrator and use it every day for half an hour.' It stimulated my juices—and kept me from drying up. Now I can enjoy intercourse with my new guy." The women in the group were curious about how she bought her vibrator. "I parked around the corner [from Eve's Garden] and wore dark glasses. Once I got in there, the young salesgirl asked if she could help. I said, 'Look, I could lie and say this is for a friend, a gag gift or something, but it's not—it's for me.' Luckily there was no one else in the store. She was very helpful. That's where I got 'The Tongue.' It's like oral sex; some women like that."

At the end of the evening, several women in their mid-70s gathered around the hostess's phonebook to find the address of the nearest shop that sold sex aids. They planned a field trip. They were looking for "The Tongue."

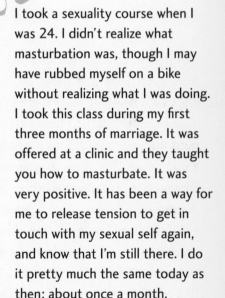

I took a sexuality course when I was 24. I didn't realize what masturbation was, though I may have rubbed myself on a bike without realizing what I was doing. I took this class during my first three months of marriage. It was offered at a clinic and they taught you how to masturbate. It was very positive. It has been a way for me to release tension to get in touch with my sexual self again, and know that I'm still there. I do it pretty much the same today as then: about once a month.

—*Denise, 55, married 26 years, Salem, Oregon*

> Well I was truly introduced to that [masturbation] when I was about 31 and I thought 'hey this feels good!'
>
> —*Bridget, 64, Detroit, Michigan*

While many women enjoy using vibrators and/or dildos, there are those who don't. Take Marla for example. She's a 63-year-old, single choir director from Mississippi who said, "I really think of it (masturbation) like eating and breathing, really essential to my life. I still do it the same way I did it when I was a little girl; I've never used a vibrator. When I've tried to do it different ways it's like I lose interest really fast and I revert back to the way I did it when I was a little girl. It's so interesting to me. It really connects me with my past too, I think."

Personal Preferences

Some women find that masturbation is as pleasurable as it has always been, but they just don't do it as often. "I think it's been great; I mean it's helped a lot," says Esther, a 70-year-old grandmother from Connecticut. "When I get horny, I masturbate and I relax and I sleep well. I realize that I do it a lot less frequently now. I used to do it a lot more often. Now on average, once every three or four weeks—it changes. It seems when I go on vacation and relax, I may masturbate more."

For many women, the decrease in frequency of masturbation seems to correlate with a general decrease in sexual desire; others connect such a reduction with more global changes in themselves. "I probably do it less now; there have been times when it's kept me from going nuts, because I wasn't getting it any other way. It's a nice way to relax in the evening when there's nothing else to do," says Judith, a 53-year-old who lives in the District of Columbia.

"I think it's less frequent 'cause I'm more comfortable in my sexual activity with my husband. I'm much more confident, less put on the spot, less pissed off, and feel better about myself," wrote Janie, a 60-year-old graphic designer who has been married to her current husband for 15 years.

Vera, a 61-year-old New Haven translator, said, "It's almost gotten nonexistent as I've gotten older—and it never was a big part of my life—partly it's because I really didn't know much about it and I really didn't know about it as a resource. I never really learned how to masturbate—it wasn't really satisfying and so it hasn't been important in at least the last ten years or so."

> I don't do it with the frequency that I used to, but every now and then I think, oh god, that would be nice. I know when I was younger I never did. But now it satisfies me when I need to be satisfied.
>
> —*Jane, 68, thrice-married, currently single, Athens, Georgia*

Women handle growing older with imaginative energy. When it comes to accommodating the limitations age can place on the body, Simone, at 52, had already planned for her "retirement":

"I would say I do it [masturbate] maybe five times out of the year, maybe more; it depends on what's happening in my life. My favorite way of self-stimulation is my hand-held shower nozzle. It's non-invasive, doesn't have to include the family members, convenient, simple. I've thought about this; I think that as I get older I'll get a chair in my shower!"

Masturbation is one way women can take control over their own sexual desire and maintain a sense of personal power. They do not need to rely exclusively on the attentions of a partner to fulfill their sexual needs. Self-pleasuring can provide the tens of millions of us over 50 with reliable, safe, and unencumbered satisfaction. It may help us reconnect with our inner selves.

It has changed in that, if it is a feeling that is coming over me and something that I want to do, I don't talk myself out of it. I think it is just that I'm getting to know me and not sublimating those feelings.

—Nancy, 58, recently left an abusive marriage Concord, New Hampshire

For example, 52-year-old Rosa, who lives in an historic section of Albuquerque, New Mexico, said, "I would say that it opened up a lot of my sexuality to me that I was not aware of. I had a male partner who introduced me to a lot of things...I thought he had to be the one. I thought, but I was wrong. So today it [masturbation] is something I engage in occasionally. Every so often you've got to make sure that you're still there."

There Are Lots of Ways to Do It

Whether you've been enjoying the pleasures of masturbating since childhood or have only recently added self-pleasuring to your to-do list, you may be curious to learn even more about the benefits. As Cathy Winks and Anne Semans mention in *The Good Vibrations Guide to Sex,* "There's no time like the present to improve your own technique." There are scores of resources including books, videos, and even websites about masturbation. Many are aimed exclusively at women. You might find it helpful to consult one of Joani Blank's many books on sexuality, such as the *Complete Guide to Vibrators,* which has detailed information about different styles of vibrators and suggestions about choosing one. Or visit a website called www. clitical.com. This cheery site contains stories, tips and techniques, product reviews, and even a place to share your own masturbation tale. Warning: the site is explicit...and it doesn't come in a plain brown wrapper.

If you are a technophobe—the kind who relies on your neighbor's teenage son to program your cell phone or your DVD player or hook up your computer—you're certainly not alone. But vibrators are a type of technology that many mature women are curious about and are quite comfortable using. Women may have heard from their daughters or nieces about a new kind of Tupperware-style party—one where attendees can buy sex toys. Or just like the women we visited with in New Jersey, they may be curious about visiting a sex

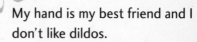

> My hand is my best friend and I don't like dildos.
> —*Shannon, 70, Trenton, New Jersey*

toy shop to learn about the ins and outs of vibrators and dildos. We've had scores of women ask us if we could escort them to such an establishment. Because we can't accompany all our readers to such a place, we'd like to describe our field trip to Babeland (formerly Toys in Babeland), a sex boutique in Seattle, to give you an idea of what you'll experience if you decide to venture out on your own. If you do decide to explore this shopping environment, consider going with a friend or taking your partner. If nothing else, the stimulation such a shared experience will give to your conversation will be worth the trip.

You can erase that picture you may have in your head of the sleazy porn shop where you would never be caught dead. Feminist sex boutiques are run by women and cater to us, though men do shop there as well. They are clean, well lighted, and comfortable. We can thank Joani Blank for starting the first such shop, Good Vibrations, in San Francisco in 1977.

Walking through the door of a shop such as the one we visited—where more than 300 sex toys are colorfully displayed—can initially be a jolt to your system. But we discovered that the ambiance was upbeat and playful. The young saleswomen were extremely knowledgeable and incredibly nonjudgmental. We learned that the variety of vibrators and dildos (those that are intended for penetration and usually don't vibrate) is enormous.

For a first time-buyer, the selection can be a bit overwhelming, so it might be helpful to have a checklist of considerations. Approach this kind of like you would when buying a car—there is no vibrator that's best for everyone, and some people still really do prefer a manual transmission!

Some considerations for buying a vibrator:

Is noise a factor? Do you live with others or in a thin-walled apartment where the hum of a vibrator might be an embarrassment? Some styles are definitely quieter than others.

Are you someone who prefers a zingy feel to a rumbly feel? Did you have trouble adjusting to your electric toothbrush because the vibration was too much? The type of vibration delivered varies from model to model. Maybe you don't want any vibration; if so, take a look at the dildos.

Find out how to clean the one you like before you buy it. Most of them cannot be put in the dishwasher!

Are you latex sensitive? You'll want to examine the wide range of materials.

Color is always a consideration. We saw some with flowers and others with swirls. The red one is out there, so is the silver one, which might even be mistaken for a hairdryer if you don't look closely!

Actually seeing and holding various styles might be the best way to find a vibrator that will answer your personal needs. However, for those who don't live near one of the boutiques or can't imagine going into one, check out the Internet...a nice alternative.

Masturbation can be an awkward topic. Our society, our faith-based institutions, and our legislators have created a negative image of masturbation, equating it with sin and immature sexuality. Women over 50 are ready to ignore the proscriptions of their childhood and are curious to explore the subject. Some were initially reluctant to talk aloud about what role, if any, masturbation had played in maintaining their sense of themselves as sexual beings—but once the ice was broken, they told us how it has been a primary element in

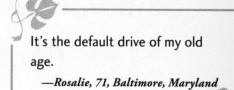

It's the default drive of my old age.

—*Rosalie, 71, Baltimore, Maryland*

maintaining positive sexual self-esteem. A large percentage of women beyond 50 have no partner, and these women say that self-pleasuring gives them sexual vivaciousness. Others use masturbation to provide new stimulation to a maturing sexual relationship or to bring themselves to orgasm when they find their sexual desire is out of sync with their partner's. As our bodies age, our sensitivity to sexual touch changes. Through self-pleasuring, women can get direct information about what feels good now, what is stimulating, and what is uncomfortable. This knowledge gives us increased control over our sexual selves—we can choose to share it with a partner or use it to enhance our personal experience. Masturbation can be an aid in healing and in maintaining a healthy vagina. As many women told us, this is a great way to increase vitality and to know that you are sexually alive. And it's certainly more fun than taking your daily multivitamin!

Many women who have never masturbated are now interested in what self-pleasuring may have to offer them. These are the women who have come to our seminars and workshops with questions about how to buy a vibrator, what kind of lubricant is best, and which shops offer dildos appropriate for older vaginas.

Evie probably said it best, "This is just for you. It's safe and fun and not nasty at all."

Truth #6

Same-Sex Relationships Don't Scare Older Women

When Women Are Attracted to Other Women After 50, They May Take A Road Less Traveled

The party was over. Ellen's many friends had gathered to reminisce with her about the days before the big Five-O and to welcome her to the informal sorority of reluctant members of AARP. Now she was sitting amidst the party detritus—crinkled paper and ribbon were scattered across the carpet, soggy streamers dangled from the hall light fixture, and her kitchen counters were strewn with leftovers. She really should let the dog out and find the Wine Away before the cabernet spots ruined her best tablecloth. But she couldn't move. Had she really told her friend Cindy that she'd love to have dinner with her again on Saturday? And what was so unusual about that anyway? For almost fifteen years, they'd been gabbing to each other regularly. They'd spent endless Saturdays shivering together on the sidelines while watching the kids play soccer, grumbled disappointedly to each other about the results of the last mayoral race, and had even confided embarrassing tales of stress incontinence in recent years.

Yet there was something about their relationship that had shifted. Since Ellen and Steve had split, she had begun spending a lot more time with Cindy, and lately the air was charged with something unsaid. Over the past six months, every time she and Cindy got together Ellen had been fantasizing about kissing her...and wondered what it would be like to touch her breasts. What was that all about?

These thoughts were new to Ellen—sex with a woman hadn't even crossed her mind until very recently. Although she and Steve had fought over finances and child rearing and home remodeling projects during the course of their twenty-two-year marriage, she'd pretty much enjoyed their sexual relationship. Dating after the demise of their marriage hadn't been the agony many of her friends had vividly decried, but there was certainly no lusty magnetism drawing her to anyone new. Not until the last six months or so. The only problem was—it wasn't a man but another woman who was sparking her interest.

She was definitely confused and conflicted. Was she just going through a phase? Could she possibly be a lesbian? Or maybe she was bisexual? How, after all these years of feeling sexual desire for men, could that desire have flipped upon itself? If it had, what would become of her? Weren't her 50s supposed to be a time for clear-eyed wisdom? She wasn't feeling particularly astute at the moment. And putting her own bewilderment aside, what would her son, who had just gotten married to the love of his life, think if he learned that his mother had a female lover?

Ellen's story reflects the reality that same-sex relationships are intriguing to a large percentage of older women. But this is certainly not a topic that women beyond 50 find easy to discuss. While quite a few participants in our study were curious about or had experimented with sex with other women, they had rarely spoken about this hidden part of their sex lives. And it's not surprising they've been silent. The debate about homosexuality raging in voting booths, churches, homes, and bedrooms across the United States today is enough to keep even the most assertive of women quiet.

Our homophobic culture can easily inhibit older women from identifying themselves as lesbian or bisexual. It's never been an easy path to walk. Even during 1970s, when the second wave of women's liberation gained influence, there were not many openly gay or bisexual women. Today, young actors and actresses may talk cavalierly about their same-sex relationships, and "pink TV" shows may focus on openly gay characters, but for older bisexual women and lesbians, passing as straight remains the common choice. It's far less provocative for an older lesbian couple to refer to themselves as roommates or friends than to label themselves as lovers.

But even nonsexual relationships between women can be multilayered. Like Ellen, numerous women we've talked to described their friendships with other women as profoundly important. Few had even considered having a same-sex relationship at earlier points in their lives. Now that they are past 50 and have more time for reflection, some have found these relationships are becoming more complicated. Some wonder if the closeness they felt might extend to the sexual realm. Maureen, a retired middle school teacher in her late 50s from Indiana, took several deep breaths and told us, "I now have gentle fantasies about women because they are gentle and know gentle touching, and probably know more about arousal."

An Unspoken truth

Our research reveals that the number of older women who live openly bisexual or gay lifestyles is only a fraction of the much larger number who find the idea of same-sex relationships appealing.

We heard similar sentiments from women across the nation whose ages spanned the decades from 50 to 90. A mature woman struggling to define her sexual identity is not an isolated phenomenon. We heard about it during discussions with women of color in L.A., older Jewish women in New Jersey, and professional women who live on the North Dakota plains.

Sexual Orientation Can Be Puzzling

There isn't, and may never be, an official tally of gays, lesbians, bisexuals, and transgendered people in the United States. (As a matter of fact, there probably isn't a good count of heterosexuals, either.) In a national survey conducted by Sell et al. in the 1990s, nearly 18 percent of U.S. women reported either homosexual attraction or behavior since age 15. The same study found that 3.6 percent of women in the United States reported they had had sex with another woman in the past five years. Another study (Laumann et al.) estimates that between 1.4 percent and 4.3 percent of women in the United States are lesbian or bisexual. Nearly 7 percent of women who responded to our survey identified themselves as bisexual and/or lesbian. Among the women we interviewed in depth, 17 percent described themselves as lesbians or bisexual; all of these women had had at least one male sexual partner at some point in her life. Based on our interviews, we also know that many women who are erotically aroused by other women did not report this fact when completing our

> There are really not two genders—there are many. There's such a variety of attraction—from the most feminine female to the most masculine man—even within same sex couples.
>
> —*Ruby, 53, Palo Alto, California*

survey. They may feel attracted to other women, but their behavior is conventionally heterosexual.

Sexual attraction to other women is not only hard to talk about, it's hard to acknowledge, even to ourselves. In *The Good Vibrations Guide to Sex,* Cathy Winks and Anne Semans write, "Sexual identity involves so much more than anatomy, and sexual expression is not controlled by biology alone—after all, we aren't uniformly hard-wired to insert tab A into slot B and call that satisfying sex. Each individual's sexuality is shaped and mediated by cultural values and expectations. And the social construct that has the greatest influence on our experience of sex is gender. Gender is a human construct, and as such, it exists on a continuum that reflects the variety of human experience."

> I find women attractive, but I don't typically have sexual relations with them. I experimented on one occasion…the woman became obsessed with me…it was awful. I decided I didn't want to be having sex with her anymore. To be honest, I don't think I particularly desired this woman. It was just an experiment. I still like to look at women. I think they are very attractive.
>
> —*Maureen, 60, Presbyterian, Cape Cod, Massachusetts*

Many of the women in our study would identify strongly with Elsie, a 75-year-old from Boston, who said, "When I think about sexual desire, it is much more about the other human being, not whether they are male or female." Elsie's comment illustrates the fact that there can be wide variations in how women think about their sexual orientation. While some women in our study would label themselves as definitely heterosexual and others would classify themselves as definitely lesbian, many have given up on categorizing and just enjoy their partners, regardless of gender and the accompanying genitalia. We came to appreciate that a woman's preference for sexual partners of one gender or the other can be as fluid as the tide: not only does desire ebb and flow over the last five decades of life, but so can sexual orientation.

One End of the Spectrum

Many women doubt they could ever become sexually intimate with another woman but understand how others find the idea appealing. Hattie, a 60-year-old from the Southwest, told us, "I think a big reason why women have lesbian relationships is that as women, you're more on the same wavelength. But I'm not interested in having a physical relationship with another woman. I've thought about it a lot, because I have a lot of friends who are lesbians, but it doesn't appeal to me. I don't want to go there, because I think it would be too much work. It would be a whole shift, a lifestyle shift, a mental shift. But I can understand it."

Although her perspective is now similar to Hattie's, Cassandra, a 59-year-old financial planner, has struggled to come to terms with two women who severely challenged her values. "I can understand how some women can be married and then happen to fall in love with a woman after a divorce. I have a friend, a nurse who was married, got divorced, and dated a lot. And now she's living with a woman and it looks like it's maybe a little more than a friendship. And I can see how women would gravitate to women. I could certainly see that happening because as we age, there just isn't that large of a pool of eligible men out there. The men die; they're impotent; they have other health problems. But at the point where it would turn sexual, I just don't know."

Cassandra went on to describe how distressed she became when two women "came on" to her. She was uncomfortable with their behavior because it was not what she expected of them, and it felt disrespectful. "After my divorce, three women friends and I (all newly single) went to Europe together. We would change roommates whenever we got to a new town. We checked in, and Sally, my 'new' roommate took a shower. Then, I did. When I came back into the room, she had posed herself on the chaise lounge wearing only her bra and pants. I thought, 'What is this all about?' She was being very suggestive, and I was so embarrassed. I just ignored her and went to bed. Then, she came to bed and took off her robe and said, 'I always sleep naked.' I was shocked. This was a woman I'd known for about a year, and I had absolutely no indication that she was bisexual or lesbian. Evidently, something about me turned her on.

"When the four of us arrived in the next town, we changed roommates again. I told my new roommate Bonnie what had happened. She started laughing. Then, Bonnie started coming on to me. Maybe Bonnie and Sally were lovers. It was so strange for me. Eventually, I couldn't take the strain. They were both fighting over me. And then, Bonnie kind of eased me out of the 'foursome'—it was almost like she was a scorned lover. The others continued to do things together but didn't include me."

For someone like Cassandra, who places herself squarely on the heterosexual side of the sexual-orientation continuum, it can be hard to understand how other women can move across the range so readily. In the search for an explanation she could relate to, Cassandra rationalized that Bonnie and Sally had attempted to meet society's expectations when they married men. She saw them as lesbians who had tried to "pass" but found that a heterosexual life didn't work for them. This may have been true, but it also may have been that the sexual desire Bonnie and Sally felt for women was just different from what they felt for men.

Moving Across the Spectrum

"Sexual desire depends on and is connected and inseparable from what attracts you to your partner," says Beth. "If your soul gets full being around a certain person it builds strong attraction. Sexual desire can be physical, but it is also spiritual, emotional, and mental as well. Look out! Because it can happen with either a man or a woman."

Cathy is 54 and works in a women's boutique in New Hampshire where she's lived since she left her husband. Today she calls herself a bisexual. She thought of herself as heterosexual prior to age 50 but acknowledges she probably wasn't truly aware of her range of options. Cathy grew up in Iowa. Her mom went to Mass every day, and Cathy herself attended Catholic schools. Her religious perspective has shifted as she's aged; on our survey, she identified herself as a Christian Buddhist. Divorced for 12 years, she has three grown children and six grandchildren. Cathy has had eight sexual partners over her lifetime; half of them have been women.

"There is a difference for me. There is definitely an emotional difference. When I am in a sexual relationship with a woman, I am much more of who I am than when I am in a sexual relationship with a man. I'm much more concerned about how I present when I'm with a man. With a woman, I'm just there and present. But when I'm with a man, I'm really concerned about how I look, how my body looks. It's more of an external focus rather than an internal one. I do feel more myself when I'm with a woman. I feel freer.

"However, I don't think there is a difference as far as the relationship per se. I can remember the first time I was with a woman I thought it was *the* answer. And what I realized is that relationships are relationships; it doesn't matter what sex your partner is. When I think about sexual desire now most of the time it relates to another human being not whether they are male or female."

Many of our interviewees echoed Cathy's feeling that it was the human connection between two people, regardless of sex, for which they yearned. Yvonne, a divorced, bisexual woman from Cherry Hill, Pennsylvania, said, "Some researcher did a profile of lesbian and bisexual women compared to heterosexual women. They discovered that although the stereotype is that lesbians and bis are always very sexual, they might in fact have less sex than heterosexual women." She further elaborated "Part of the thing of straight women having sex is that sometimes when you're with a man, the only time you have closeness is when you're having sex. When you're with a woman, in general, you get a lot of your closeness by cuddling and the focus is not on having sex but of being close."

Yvonne's statement resonated with many of the women we've encountered. Feeling closer to her partner led her to a greater depth of intimacy. She knew she could express her deepest thoughts and feelings. And through this intimacy she became more convinced that the path she has chosen was one that allowed her to "speak my truth and feel good about my actions." With all the negative messages our society gives about same-sex relationships, the positive sexual self-esteem Yvonne's relationship offers is a powerful gift.

The Other End of the Spectrum

While Yvonne describes herself a bisexual, Maxine, who has had two long-term relationships, one with a man to whom she was married for ten years and one for nine years with a woman, sees herself as a lesbian. Maxine told us she's had about twenty-five sexual partners of both sexes, although she's been predominately with women.

"Probably I recognized that I was a lesbian when I was a teenager, maybe even before. I didn't know any lesbians at the time. I remember going to the library to look up the word *homosexual*. The psychiatrist's manual said it was some sort of deviation. And I remember thinking, 'I don't feel deviant. I feel normal.' What I feel for some of my girlfriends is a pure feeling of love or maybe lust, but I never accepted it as a deviance.

"I thought my family would disown me if I told them about my sexual preferences, so I got married. I met Arnie at the beginning of my senior year in high school. We dated for four years and then married. We waited for three year to have kids.

"I was an idealistic person when I got married. Even though we dated for four years, we didn't actually have sex until a week before we got married. I wanted save myself for my marriage. I guess that sounds kind of silly. I remember after we had sex I was thinking, 'Is that all there is? I could have waited one more week for that!' And then, because I waited, I was really looking forward to having sex when I was married.

"Prior to marriage, he was always after me to have sex. And I always said, 'no.' After we married, I was the one who was free to enjoy sex. He would stay up really late and watch Johnny Carson. I could wear a negligee or even nothing. It wouldn't interest him at all. It made me feel bad about myself. 'What was wrong with me? He wanted me, and now he doesn't.' It probably was the conquest or something.

"The beginning of the end was when my second baby was born. She had some medical problems and almost died. Arnie refused to take off from work to go with me to an endocrinologist. I've never forgiven him for that. I had to face our daughter's illness all by myself. If he had gone with me, I probably would still be married to him even though I love women. What made me divorce him and try my wings as a lesbian actually had nothing to do with my being a lesbian . . . It had more do with him being unemotional and insensitive. I was in an emotional vacuum and craved more.

"I know I'm not just attracted to a body type, because I've been with all different kinds of bodies. Having sexual desire for another person is very much linked with what they do and how they are. For example, if a person is an activist, that really turns me on. I'm not attracted to 'lipstick lesbians,' because I want to see the real person, not someone with a mask on." There's little ambiguity in Maxine's

An Unspoken Truth

When I'm with men I do more fantasizing. When I'm with a woman I don't need to and I get more aroused from the experience. There is a way that I'm in my body differently.

—Jamie, 58, Sarasota, Florida

sexual orientation now, and she's looking forward to sharing her life with a woman who also shares her viewpoint.

After two marriages, one child, and a couple of other same-sex relationships, Angie, a 53-year-old X-ray technician from Boise, Idaho, says she's found her life partner—another woman. "When I was in heterosexual relationships, there were parts of me the men didn't have a clue about. Now, so much of who my lover and I are when we're together is more similar—and somehow more wholesome."

When asked why, at midlife, she's chosen to identify herself as a lesbian, Angie told us, "It's really all about the relationship, about having a companion who shares my interests and about our similarities as women. But I'd be lying if I said it wasn't also about our sexual chemistry too."

Is the Quality of Desire Different?

What happens to their sexual desire when women switch from totally heterosexual relationships to same-sex ones? Is depth of desire dependent on the gender of the person they're involved with, or is it tied more to the relationships? Is the level or intensity of desire the same or different when they have a lover who is a woman?

Interviewees and participants in discussion groups repeatedly mentioned how comfortable they feel with other women. Wanda, 71, said, "When I'm with a woman there is a sense of being known, and knowing the other person in a way that you just don't have with a man." But when asked if their desire is different, the responses vary quite markedly.

One perspective is offered by Rachel, a Rhode Islander in her mid-50s who currently lives on the West Coast. Rachel acknowledged that she has had many sexual partners in her lifetime. Divorced at 22, she considered herself a lesbian for 25 years. Now, she thinks of herself as bisexual and has had a male lover, Henry, for the past two and a half years—and relishes the relationship.

"Sexual desire has always been important to my health and well-being. It is very important for me now, in my relationship with Henry, and it was very important for many years when my partner was a woman for whom sex was difficult. Desire went on a back burner with her but it never went away for me. Now I don't know if it's some sort of new freedom or making up for lost time, or having a lover who really enjoys sex and no children at home and having the time and attention."

When asked if the quality of her desire was different when she is with a woman rather than with a man, Rachel says, "I would and wouldn't attribute the differences in desire to gender. It really depends on who I'm in love with and partnering with. My sexual desire definitely plays off the other person. With my former (woman) partner, sex was such an issue; my desire went away out of self-preservation. Henry really enjoys sex a lot. We're very compatible and often comment, 'We've certainly met our match!' Perhaps the element of a long-term relationship—in a relationship with a woman, sex becomes less and less important. So it really doesn't seem to be gender related—it's person related."

Q. Is the quality of your sexual desire different when you're with a woman rather than with a man?
A. The physiology is different, the energetic connection may be stronger; the relationship issues are the same.

—*Gina, 55, Alexandria, Virginia*

Rachel wonders if the experience of sexual desire and growing old together after 50 is different for heterosexual women than for lesbians and bisexuals. "Can you separate out the relationship from the sex? It's different not to have kids at home, with the accompanying responsibilities. Is it because I'm with a man? Is it because I feel in the prime of my life? I think there is something delightful about not worrying about whether I'm going to have kids, what the kids are doing, what kind of career and job I will have. I know who I am. One of the benefits of aging, I've already made family."

Rachel presents herself as totally confident and comfortable in her sexual skin, regardless of the gender of the person who is the focus of her sexual desire. "Maybe it was the water I drank growing up in Providence or something that gives me my confidence. I feel so fortunate that I can be with a man and just don't feel conflicted although I really thought I was a lesbian. I know I am a strong capable and sensuous woman. Psychologically, I'm pretty intact."

Achieving positive sexual self-esteem like Rachel has is challenging when you're a woman over 50, and for those who are grappling with questions of sexual orientation, it can be an even more complex task.

Sexual Self-Esteem and Sexual Orientation

Older women thinking about being involved in same-sex relationships tell us they often wrestle with issues of acceptance and self-worth. In some ways, they are not unlike younger women who are trying to resolve issues of sexual identity—they are just coming to their struggle 30 years later. Some continue to be closeted for self-protection while others have found it possible to come out to their families and co-workers. And many have yet to decide how or when to try a same-sex partnership. Most of them have fought at some point to quell the chorus of internal critics whose noisy voices intrude upon an otherwise peaceful life.

Frequently women described being fearful about how the rest of the world might view them. Michelle, a 55-year-old self-described bisexual, said, "I grew up with my older sister and two brothers in New Orleans and went to Catholic schools until the tenth grade. (I

The Missing Ladle

Anna invited her 80-year-old mother over for dinner. During the meal, her mother just couldn't help noticing how attentive Anna's roommate was. She had become curious about her recently divorced daughter's sexuality, and this only made her more so. Over the course of the evening, while watching the two women interact, she started to wonder if there was more between Anna and her roommate than met the eye. Reading her mother's thoughts, Anna volunteered, "I know what you must be thinking, Mother, but I assure you, Dorothy and I are just roommates."

A week later, Dorothy came to Anna and said, "Ever since your mother came to dinner, I've been unable to find the beautiful silver gravy ladle. You don't suppose she took it, do you?"

Anna said, "Well, I doubt it, but I'll e-mail her just to be sure."

So she sat down at the computer and wrote, "Dear Mother, I'm not saying you 'did' take a gravy ladle from my house, and I'm not saying that you 'did not' take a gravy ladle. But the fact remains that one has been missing ever since you were here for dinner."

The next day, Anna opened an e-mail from her mother that read, "Dear Daughter, I'm not saying that you 'do' sleep with Dorothy, and I'm not saying that you 'do not' sleep with Dorothy. But the fact remains that if she was sleeping in her own bed, she would have found the gravy ladle by now."

was kicked out in the fourth grade for a while, as the priests didn't think my father tithed enough.) When I began to date, I was sexually attracted to anyone who was attracted to me. I didn't really choose the person—I didn't choose for my soul; instead, I chose for my fears—insecurity, lack of money."

Shame and embarrassment can have a withering effect on self-esteem. In an effort to avoid such painful feelings, many women resisted the draw to act on their sexual desires. For example, Wylene, a highly respected 59-year-old chief information officer from the East Coast, who has been married for more than 30 years, told us about her struggle for self-acceptance in light of some of the sexual choices she's made. "My first sexual relationships were with girls. The thing about my sexuality was that I didn't feel like I was OK; there was something wrong with me. I was with women, but I couldn't enjoy my sexuality. This whole issue has been really confusing to me, but I feel like I've resolved it and I can live with it. Sometimes I think I'm really a lesbian but that I happen to be in love with this man. And I guess deep down I feel like it's more acceptable from a societal viewpoint to be with him."

Other women fear that trying a same-sex relationship could mar their familial relationships. Sarah, a Jewish widow in her mid-70s who lives near Miami Beach, worries about the criticism and rejection she might face if she acted on her feelings. She told us, "I love my women friends. We do everything together. The only reason I don't act on my attraction to women now is that I don't want to have to listen to what my kids (who are 48 and 49 respectively) will say about it!" Sarah simply didn't want to deal with the consequences of following through on her inclinations and so chose to remain celibate. Although she was willing to express her thoughts to us, she doubts she could feel really good about herself if she took a woman lover. Restructuring old emotional ties and sexual impulses and becoming more open to possibilities can be liberating for many women, but not for Sarah.

Other women say the effect of our ageist society on our psyches is enough to deal with without having to also agonize over sexual-preference issues. For example, Lucy, a 72-year-old grandmother from Louisiana, told us, "I'm already aware that I'm treated as a 'sweet little old lady.' I'm not now, and never have been sweet; I'm just older now. I don't want to add to my problems. The other day I went to see a new doctor. First I had to complete the form that asks if I'm married or single. Then, my doctor asked if I was sexually active. I began to wonder what it would be like to tell her that I'm thinking about becoming sexually involved with another woman. I certainly wasn't willing to mention that to her. It's really too much of a hassle to go through all of this. It's not worth it."

Then there were those women who decided they were willing to take a risk and explore same-sex relationships. They discovered that acknowledging their sexual attraction toward women considerably heightened their congruency quotient. Feeling they had finally achieved a sense of control over an important part of their lives meant they had a newfound sense of self-worth, and they were able to refill a depleted portion of their spirit.

As a teenager, Angie thought sexual desire was only a physical response, and one that was always initiated by a male. She really didn't understand her own sexual desire, nor did she realize that she could have control over it. In her previous relationships, even if she did have the desire, she didn't act on it. "This went on well into my life and in all of my heterosexual relationships, even in both of my marriages. When I recognized (and acted upon) my attraction to women, I felt on a more equal playing field and could express my desire more readily. It definitely has something to do with equal power.

"The first time I was sexually active was in high school…for two years. In 1970, I moved to New York City and ended up breaking my fiancé's pea-pickin' little heart when I broke our engagement.

It was also in New York where I met my first husband. I got pregnant and we ended up staying married for seven years.

"Becoming acquainted with some lesbians in the mid-1970s began to push my personal boundaries, so I guess the seed was planted then. I never thought or considered myself a potential lesbian. In fact, even now I don't even like that word. I'd much rather just say that I'm in a relationship with another woman. Yet even then I knew I was always more comfortable and relaxed around women. In my early 30s I went to Europe for three months and decided that I did want to be in a relationship. I even considered the possibility that I might fall in love with a women as I figured it doesn't matter which sex you're in a relationship with. When I returned to the United States, I fell back into my old patterns and got into a relationship with the man who became my second husband, a marriage that lasted twelve years.

"I craved a healthy relationship, and for some reason I didn't see that as possible with a man. Then, right before I turned 50, I just didn't care what other people thought. When I was in a committed relationship with my second husband, I just didn't let my mind go there. In fact, I didn't even want to be sexual with a woman. I was drawn to women but didn't feel sexual desire. Catholics just don't do those things!

"Now, I'm aware of my own desire because I feel it's so much more natural. I'm attracted to every part of who my partner is—that desire is not for sex, it's a desire for being in her presence. The sexual desire is great—it's more fun, more giving, more intense. We have sex about two to three times per week—and that's not really any different than the number of times I had sex with my second husband, but the satisfaction and the equalness and the intimacy has a 'whole person' aspect."

Other women found that satisfying their sexual needs by being with a woman has become a necessary condition for their sense of

well-being. Tanya is one such woman. "In my 40s, living unpartnered for the first time in many years, a grace descended upon me. I
began to recognize my own lovability. Despite the broken relationships, the elusive and dramatic sexual peaks and crashes, despite the
30-year divorce from my own wholeness, I was indeed worthy. In
truth, I fell in love with myself. The rest is relatively predictable and
miraculous nonetheless. A woman appeared in my life for whom I
felt passion and with whom I shared countless values. I didn't have
a list, but if I had, she would have matched it perfectly. One step
at a time, my sexual desire became rooted in choice rather than
survival.

"Fourteen years later and in our mid-50s, we are still exploring
our partnership. I don't call it a 'sexual partnership,' although it is,
but the sex is not what defines it. It's there, in the background, available when invited. Since sex is no longer the source of enormous
highs and lows, it's no longer the cord I require to graft me back
together. It smells good and makes me laugh. It's neither regular nor
predictable, and it no longer has a desperate element. It's optional
and less complicated. Most of the time, I can't even remember what
all the fuss was about."

Searching for Some Answers

Moving beyond the traditional sexual script our culture has written
for older women can be quite overwhelming, especially for those
who thought they had put questions of sexual identity to bed years
earlier. Mature women who find themselves attracted to other
women can feel that they are entering a whole new world. They are
often baffled because they don't know where to turn or are uncer-
tain about how to learn more. If you or a friend is struggling to find
your way, to gain a better understanding of your feelings, or if you

just want to find out more about rejecting or initiating same-sex relationships, we offer the following suggestions:

1. Get informed

- Visit an independent and/or woman-owned book store. Most
  offer a safe, quiet place to peruse the shelves and are more apt
  to offer a wide range of books and reading materials geared to
  questions of sexual identity and behavior. Reading about other
  women's experiences while you are engaged in personal soul-
  searching and exploration can be enlightening.

- Search the Internet. Two organizations—the American Society
  of Aging (www.asaging.org/networks/LGAIN) and SIECUS,
  the Sexuality Information and Education Council of the
  United States (www.siecus.org/pubs/biblio)—have websites
  that offer wonderful lists with helpful materials and good resources for straight, lesbian, gay, bisexual, and transgendered
  people.

  Another website with a list of resources is Older Lesbians
  Organizing for Change (www.oloc.org). The organization en-
  courages women to confront ageism and develops and dis-
  seminates educational materials.

  Chat lines oriented toward bisexual and lesbian women
  abound. While some are definitely geared to "women seeking
  women," others have a gentler approach and provide insight
  into the fluidity of sexual expression. Asking questions in the
  safety of your own home can be a low-risk first step.

- Take a human sexuality course. Women's studies programs at
  universities and community colleges usually offer such classes
  and sometimes give senior discounts or reduced tuition to
  women of a certain age. If the thought of sitting in a class-
  room with people half your age is too intimidating, and you're

computer savvy, try taking one of the many distance-learning courses offered.

2. Evaluate Your Own Feelings

- Start a journal. Most women experience a wide swing in emotions when they consider a big change in their lives. Keeping a record of how your feelings change can give you perspective and help you appreciate what really matters to you.

- Ask yourself some questions:

  What makes me feel best about myself as a sexual person?
  What is most important to me in a sexual relationship?
  How would I react if my sexual choices were judged negatively by others?
  How is my sexual self-esteem today? When has it been highest, what contributed to that?

- Examine your answers. Look for patterns in your history of sexual relationships. Perhaps the idea of exploring same-sex relationships will benefit your sense of sexual self-worth; perhaps not. Be honest with yourself. If you can't see your own patterns clearly (a difficult thing for most of us), consult a professional therapist—that's exactly what they are trained to help us do.

3. Talk about it

- Take the plunge and start a conversation with one or more of your women friends who you think would be open to talking about same-sex relationships. You might say something like, "The other day I was reading a book about older women's sexuality, and there were stories of women whose close friendships began to spill over into the sexual area. I can understand how that might happen, but it's still confusing to me. What do you think?" or "The younger generation seems to be more open about changing sexual orientation. I don't really know what to make of it, do you?"

- Take someone who you know has been involved in a same-sex relationship out for coffee or tea. Let them know you are curious about sexual identity. Ask them if they would mind answering some questions you have about the realities of a same-sex partnership.

- Talk to a therapist or counselor who has experience working with older women and questions of sexual identity. You may wish to consult with the American Association of Sex Educators, Counselors and Therapists (www.AASECT.org), or use the referral services offered by the American Psychological Association (www.apa.org).

- Attend a meeting of a resource group in your area. Googling bisexual resource groups, for instance, results in the names of dozens of such networks in cities all across the United States, including Seattle; San Francisco; Los Angeles; San Diego; Davis County, Utah; Chicago; Indianapolis; Austin; Houston; Richmond, Virginia; Phoenix; Birmingham, Alabama; and New York.

It used to be that the two old ladies who lived down the block or in the apartment upstairs called themselves sisters; people may have wondered, but no one ever spoke about it out loud. Today's world is more accepting of gay relationships, but the notion that a 70-year-old grandmother could be having a sexual relationship with her girlfriend is still a stretch for many people. Our culture may not be ready to openly acknowledge it, but straight women over 50 who have developed warm, caring, and intense friendships with other women do sometimes get turned on by their friends. Such a switch in sexual orientation can lead to a blossoming of sexual self-esteem or be a cause of wilting shame.

Our research has led us to see sexual orientation as existing on a continuum: the notion that there is a broad range between the most heterosexually oriented woman and the woman who is only attracted to other women. From the stories we've heard, it appears that for many older women, sexual desire is more often about the quality of the relationship, not the sex of the person who evokes the desire. Kathryn, a soft-spoken redhead from Denver, said it well, "It doesn't matter if I'm with a man or with a woman. I would like to be 85 and still be sleeping naked in bed with someone and loving my body, and feeling understood and loved."

Truth #7

Sexual Vitality Can Thrive Despite Ill Health

When Illness and Ailments Interfere, Sexual Ingenuity Steps in

Patti and Ben felt lucky. Fueled by lucrative jobs and good health, they'd been able to donate countless volunteer hours and thousands of dollars to benefit their small Midwestern community. Their two adult kids were warm and bright and productive—and they weren't likely to move back home for the foreseeable future. Their sex life had always been important to both of them and worked as the delicious glue that held them together.

Patti was in her early 60s and had just retired from her job as a bank manager when things began to change. At first she noticed that getting out of bed in the morning was becoming painful. Awakening stiff and sore, she hit on a simple solution, "Ben, let's replace that old mattress we've been sleeping on." But the new orthopedic model made no difference at all.

"I've got to start working out again," Patti thought. With high expectations, she joined the local Y; but her daily workouts didn't seem to help all that much either. One day she drove home after her yoga class and found that she could barely get out of her car. By the time Ben got home from work, the aches had abated and Patti hadn't really given them much more thought. That night, she reached for him and they began to make love. It wasn't until Ben lay on top of her that the pain returned. "Oh, my hip, Ben! You have to get off, I can't do this!"

She made an appointment with her doctor. "Well, it's osteoarthritis, I'm sure. We all get this to some degree as we age. You can take anti-inflammatory medication, and that should help."

Arthritis—damn. Both her parents had had it, and by the time they were in their 70s, they had had to quit traveling, and even the gardening had had to go. It was not the future Patti had envisioned for herself. The medications the doctor recommended upset her stomach. Then she had a bout with neck pain that triggered headaches. A MRI showed deteriorating discs in her cervical spine—this wasn't going to go away or heal itself. Getting older was no picnic.

> The spirit is willing, but because of my osteoarthritic hip, sex itself is impossible.
>
> —*Tessie, 74, a long-married North Carolinian*

And what about sex? Patti had been going to the same physician for more than thirty years, yet it was awkward for her to say anything to him about this subject. She and Ben were going to have to figure it out for themselves. Meanwhile, Ben, anxious about causing her pain, seemed to lose all interest in sex. It wasn't that he didn't desire her; it was just that every time he touched her, he felt he had to be so careful. Patti, too, worried about getting into painful positions. Yet she yearned for Ben. Though he treated her with concern, he didn't seem as warm and loving. When they first tried to talk about it, they both felt sad and a little hopeless.

Patti discovered that arthritis is a sneaky disease. Occasionally, she would wake up feeling great. Other days, she could hardly move. But regular exercise helped keep her pain and stiffness at bay, and staying fit bolstered her sexual self-esteem. As she learned more about her disease and its effect on her body, she and Ben talked more easily about the adjustments they could make in their sexual activity. She told Ben, "I miss the spontaneity in our love-making. I can't be sure that my body will always cooperate. But I don't want to give up—it means too much to me. We may not be able to do it as often as we did, but when we do it's still wonderful. We just have to take it slow. I feel like I have to make friends with this body of mine again—I'm still a sensual woman, not just an arthritis sufferer, as they say on TV."

As Patti and Ben found out, aging can bring all sorts of illnesses and ailments that require modifying our sex lives. It's easy to get disheartened when we stare into the face of old age and see the multiple signs of physical deterioration. In fact, 20 percent of the women who responded to our survey indicated that changes due to physical illness, surgery, or chronic disease had caused their sexual desire to plummet. And another 4 percent mentioned they were afraid that sexual exertion might aggravate some underlying physical condition. Quite a few bought into the myth that the aging female body loses its capacity for sexual pleasure because ill health trumps sex: if we aren't healthy we can't, and maybe shouldn't, enjoy sexual activity. Women often spoke to us about finding that their passion had evaporated in the face of pain—their own as well as their partner's. For others, the

> Arthritis makes certain positions uncomfortable. Even though my husband is impotent we still enjoy intimate contacts of several kinds: deep kisses, "naked hugs," physical touching. Occasionally, I bring myself to climax with fantasy and slight rubbing—this usually does not take very long!
>
> —*Andrea, 78, San Francisco, California*

fatigue that accompanied their sickness seemed to dampen their desire.

Yet in spite of pain, fatigue, limited mobility, surgeries, and numbing medications, women across the last five decades of life have found ways to remain connected to their sexuality. Their ardor may take a different form, their sensations may be altered, and their bodies may not look or move like they used to, but they have survived with their sexual self-esteem intact. For example, Claire, a 65-year-old retired bus driver from Pennsylvania, had endured five abdominal surgeries over the past three years. "I've been to the hospital so many times that I'm on a first-name basis with all the nurses on 4 East. I love it when they come into my room, sit on the edge of my bed, and tell me off-color jokes. It kinda makes my belly hurt, but boy do I feel better. I've never been a good joke teller, so I've taken to writing down the punch lines so I can tell them to my husband, Art, and we can giggle together. Joking around about sex reminds me that I'm a woman and that Art and I have some good sexy times ahead."

Claire also worried that Art wouldn't find her attractive anymore. "I used to have a really cute, flat stomach. For a while I was upset because I thought Art would be turned off by my weird stomach bulges. I look like someone drove a truck over me. I even asked my doctor if he couldn't do something about all the scars. He told me to talk to a plastic surgeon in a few years. When I told Art what I'd mentioned to the doctor, he thought I was crazy to even think about such a thing. He smiled and winked at me and told me that he still thought I was the sexiest thing around just the way I am!"

Regardless of the physical state of our bodies, we continue to crave touch and intimacy. Maintaining positive sexual self-worth can be a key to the healing process. We have found that older women are remarkable skilled at tapping deep into that well of creative resourcefulness that can help them meet these needs. Faced with major changes in their own health or the health of their

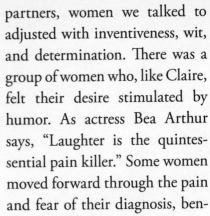

I enjoy sex more during the afternoon when I am rested, not at night when I am tired or in the morning when I need to get to work.

—*Julia, 58, Moscow, Idaho*

partners, women we talked to adjusted with inventiveness, wit, and determination. There was a group of women who, like Claire, felt their desire stimulated by humor. As actress Bea Arthur says, "Laughter is the quintessential pain killer." Some women moved forward through the pain and fear of their diagnosis, benefiting from a well-ingrained sense of sexual self-esteem. Others chose to put sex on the back burner while they gathered their strength to fight. And another group found that sexual desire simply vanished in the presence of a serious medical condition.

Chronic Diseases and Dampened Desire

Many infirmities can distract us from our ability to enjoy our sexual lives. Their impact is sometimes direct and interferes with any kind of sexual activity; other times they subtly wear away our sexual energy.

Diabetes is one of those selfish diseases that can rob its hostess of sensual pleasure. But in the hands of a resourceful woman who has been sexually oriented all her life, it is not the formidable obstacle it might otherwise be. We met Anna, who was diagnosed with diabetes five years ago, in her water-aerobics class. A powerfully inventive storyteller, she loved to regale the bevy of one-piece-only bathing-suited beauties with tales of her exploits as a military nurse and the eccentricities of her two marriages.

Anna is madly in love with her second husband, Charlie, whom she finds much sexier than her first. "He understands that I'm a sexual being and that sex is very important to me. I've finally found

Singing A New Song

Some new titles to some old tunes:

Herman's Hermits—"Mrs. Brown, You've Got a Lovely Walker"
Bobby Darin—"Splish, Splash, I Was Havin' a Flash"
The Temptations—"Papa's Got a Kidney Stone"
Marvin Gaye—"I Heard It Through the Grape-Nuts"
Procol Harem—"A Whiter Shade of Hair"
Johnny Nash—"I Can't See Clearly Now"
Paul Simon—"Fifty Ways to Lose Your Liver"
Leo Sayer—"You Make Me Feel Like Napping"
ABBA—"Denture Queen"
Roberta Flack—"The First Time Ever I Forgot Your Face"
Commodores—"Once, Twice, Three Times to the Bathroom"
The Bee Gees—"How Can You Mend a Broken Hip?"
Ringo Starr—"I Get by with a Little Help from Depends"

my sexual equal and we've found a balance together." As they move into their 80s, Anna expects that their sexual desire for one another will continue to bloom. "My only concern is maintaining my physical endurance."

She has had trouble controlling her blood sugar levels but says, "I'm not going to let a thing like this slow down my sex life." Anna and Charlie long ago learned the value of talking about their sexual needs with each other. "At first we were a bit shy about asking for what we liked. So we have some pet names for certain things, and now that we have some chronic health problems and some of those things don't feel good or work to stimulate me anymore, we can try something else." Anna admitted it took some time and considerable ingenuity, but they've figured out an approach that works for them.

"We now plan our sexual encounters around my health needs and usually have sex in the afternoon when my blood sugar is most stable. We're definitely a 'bedspread couple.'"

At times, the medical problems facing a couple can simply overwhelm them and push their sexual relationship into a different mode. This can be the case with a condition that strikes with sudden and frightening force, like heart disease or stroke. The American Heart Association (AHA) reminds us that "there's no reason why heart patients can't resume sexual activity as soon as they feel ready for it." The usual guideline given is that if you can climb four flights of stairs at an easy pace without difficulty or significant angina, you can handle the physical exertion of intercourse without a problem. After a heart attack, women often find that resuming sexual contact with their partner is a boon to their self-esteem, but it is important to take it slow and be prepared to make adjustments.

A stroke can hamper sexual expression, sensation, and response as well as general mobility. Oftentimes survivors of a stroke or heart attack are faced with making a lot of adjustments in a short span of time. Such stress can lead to confusion, irritation, and withdrawal. With all this going on, it may be tempting to dismiss low sexual interest as unimportant, but a dramatic and persistent drop in libido can be a sign of depression. It's not uncommon for patients with these conditions to experience some depression, but it is important to seek treatment if it is prolonged.

> My husband, due to medications and stroke, was not really involved in sex the last 15 to 20 years. Cuddling and touching was the limit of involvement.
>
> —*Hope, 82, Oahu, Hawaii*

Even when long-term disabilities follow a stroke or heart attack, the need for touch and affection can be met. Patience, creativity, and knowledge are all essential ingredients for rebuilding your love life. Take Vivien, who suffers from congestive heart failure. "I was about 75 when it first hit me. I was so tired all the time. I had trouble breathing when I was lying flat, so the last thing I wanted to do was to go to bed and make love. And my sexual desire was non-existent anyway. I was pretty down, but talked to my doctor and read some pamphlets. I've figured out that I just can't do some of the things I used to. My husband Elmer and I no longer have sexual intercourse, but we enjoy holding hands and hugging. We snuggle while we're watching TV, and we still tell each other how much we care. And we do laugh together—that's the best medicine."

But it's not always possible to laugh together. One of the most insidious ailments to strike older women is depression. It was Terri's total lack of interest in sex, or in anything else that used to bring her joy, that finally drove her to consult her physician. Turning 50 had coincided with a few other life-changing events that had left her numb for several months. First her father succumbed to Alzheimer's disease, which had been a cause for deep sadness as well as relief. Then her cat, who had been the one constant companion in her life for the last twelve years, was hit by a car. Divorced and living alone, Terri had found her life dramatically emptied by those two losses. Sleepless nights soon became the norm, her appetite dwindled (another event that she might have celebrated if she weren't feeling so rotten), and she had no desire to see her friends.

"When I didn't even want to have sex with Paul, my new boyfriend who I was ga-ga over, I realized that it was more than just 'the blues' and that it wasn't going to pass on its own. I went to see my doctor, who immediately recommended an antidepressant. It helped a lot. I started to sleep better and have more energy, but my sex drive didn't return." Terri's experience is very common. Most SSRIs (selective serotonin reuptake inhibitors), the class of antidepressants including Prozac and Zoloft and many others, are notorious for having "sexual side effects." They tend to inhibit sexual desire and sometimes sexual response as well. Be sure to discuss these issues with your prescriber. Research consistently shows that the most effective treatment for depression is a combination of therapy and medication. A well-trained therapist can help you evaluate the benefits of medication in light of any sexual side effects you may be experiencing and, in concert with your doctor or other practitioner, determine the best approach for you. It is usually very helpful to include your sexual partner in these discussions so his or her concerns can also be addressed.

Sexually Transmitted Diseases, Herpes, and HIV/AIDS

Those of us over 50 probably remember seeing grainy filmstrips and viewing newsreels at the movies that spoke of the untoward pain of people who were suffering from the long-term effects of gonorrhea and syphilis. Our high school and college counselors warned us about the dangers of unprotected sex and encouraged us to use condoms. But even though we've left the first five decades of our lives behind, we are still vulnerable to sexually transmitted diseases. You may have been with your partner for a long time, but what if you find out that he's been unfaithful and has been having unprotected sex? As Janine, 73, related, "After the shock of my husband's infidelity wore off, I realized the next thing I needed to do was head straight to the health department and get tested."

An Unspoken Truth

Twelve percent of women who responded to our survey were concerned about getting a sexually transmitted disease ("In these times, it pays to be celibate"); 9 percent indicated that infidelity was a major reason for fading desire.

Janine's partner had been unfaithful; others discover their partners have been involved in drug use. According to www.seniorhealth.about.com, users of drugs such as heroin "are not the only people who might share needles. People with diabetes, for example, who inject insulin or draw blood to test glucose levels, might also use the same needle. People age 50 and older may not recognize HIV symptoms in themselves because they think what they are feeling and experiencing is part of normal aging." HIV/AIDS is growing rapidly in the over-50 crowd, so before starting a new sexual relationship, be sure you and your potential partner both get tested. It's simple and easy, and just talking about the necessity to do so demonstrates that you're enthusiastic about the potential partnership and care about his or her health and well-being.

Though not fatal like HIV/AIDS, there is no cure for herpes, another sexually transmitted disease. Living with herpes can be a trial, but outbreaks of the disease can sometimes be controlled through diet, decreasing your stress level, and the use of antiviral therapy. Be sure to let any new sexual partner know if you have genital or nongenital herpes. Ask them if they have it, or if there is any chance that they have been exposed to herpes recently. Taking precautions such as avoiding skin-to-skin contact with affected areas when you have an outbreak is essential. Be sure to use latex condoms, and talk to your health-care practitioner about medications that may be helpful.

Cancer and Sex

So many of the women involved in our research were survivors of some form of cancer or had partners who were that it demands special mention. We heard how cancer can ravage a woman's sexual desires regardless of her age, her relationship status, her income level, or her religious beliefs. Sandra, a 54-year-old Latina who lives in San Jose, California, talked about "the aftereffects of cancer and a bone marrow transplant, chemo and radiation: without estrogen intercourse is very painful. The whole idea scares me." The fear of breast cancer is particularly great for older women. The 1999 statistics issued by the National Cancer Institute state that while a woman's chances of developing breast cancer by age 30 are only 1 in 2,212, by the time she is 80 her chances are 1 in 10.

With all the press about the results of the long-term Women's Health Initiative study that demonstrated a link between hormone replacement therapy and cancer, we had dozens of women in our study who told us that they had stopped taking HRT.

Gladys, who had battled breast cancer in her 50s, commented, "The changes in my desire are directly related to the aftereffects of cancer treatment. I think it's the lack of estrogen that is so devastating." At 66, she's a 9-year, grateful survivor. "All of the experience has left me with extraordinarily dry skin, dry-eye syndrome, severe back pain, and painful intercourse due to the lack of estrogen, which I can never take. Thank God that my loving, caring husband of forty-six years is totally understanding. No matter the degree of arousal, there is no moisture produced. It is a regrettable situation!! We have tried all manner of lubrication, but it just doesn't work."

> I had breast cancer five years ago and had both breasts removed followed by reconstruction. Because I can't take HRT I don't have much sexual desire and sex is painful. I miss that part of our relationship and feel it has been a negative influence in our marriage.
>
> —*Sharon, 54, Taos, New Mexico*

In a 2002 study published in the *Journal of the National Cancer Institute,* Dr. Patricia Ganz and her colleagues found that five years after being diagnosed with breast cancer, women who were no longer taking any medications other than Tamoxifen reported "no change in sexual interest or in the frequency of reporting pain with intercourse (from what had been reported at the time of the diagnosis). The increased symptoms and sexual problems reported in these survivors are associated with aging in normal healthy women." Many women in our study, however, felt that changes in their sexual desire were an indirect consequence of their breast cancer. For example, Heidi, a 57-year-old mother of three in Columbus, Ohio, told us that she still has occasional feelings of desire but rarely acts on them. "Breast cancer forced me to go off hormones and this created many problems. Tamoxifen aggravated the hormonal loss. I also have severe cervical spinal stenosis, so positioning is often difficult and painful."

We met Sherry, a handsome woman in her early 60s, at a house gathering in the Southwest. She's never married. Sherry still hopes to meet a man with whom she could form a long-term relationship, but cancer treatment has made sexual intimacy a much lower priority. "I was diagnosed with breast cancer in 1993; after going through chemotherapy, I lost most of the desire for sex. Plus I haven't found a partner to suit my taste. The ones I attract are all too young (20s and 30s). I want a man at least in his 50s or 60s."

When medications used to treat a life-threatening illness, like cancer, have side effects—a reduction in sexual desire, vaginal dryness, irritability, and increased fatigue—many women do decide that penetrative sex is no longer worth it. Sally is a woman on Tamoxifen who has made this decision: "I had a breast biopsy a couple of years ago that showed not a cancer, but some abnormal cells, that had to be followed up; it's called LCIS. And so I'm on Tamoxifen and within six months or so it's become quite painful—like when I have a pelvic exam and the doctor puts in the speculum it really hurts. I'm dry and I think the tissue has gotten thinner. My husband and I haven't had partner sex in six months or more, probably more, and I know it would hurt. It did hurt the last couple of times, you know. So I don't think I'm interested in partner sex at all, between my vibrator, and Tamoxifen, and my husband not being able to perform real well himself."

There are women who have battled cancer, some more than once, and have come out the other side with an increased appreciation for intimacy and the pleasure of human touch. Barbara is one of those women. Her story demonstrates how letting go of expectations and allowing yourself to enjoy your gifts can help you reframe your life experience.

After surviving a battle with breast cancer in her 30s, Barbara's marriage began to fizzle. "I think my illness was a part of it. I knew things weren't good between us, and then when I had to face my mortality I realized we just didn't have what it takes to make it." She divorced, and for the next 12 years concentrated on raising her daughter on her own. Her work as a teacher and the challenges of parenting filled her life. She dated some but had no serious relationships. It was during that 12-year stretch that she fell ill and was once again diagnosed with cancer. Overcoming the "big C" a second time had a profound effect on her. "I am not afraid anymore. I used to be kind of, I don't know, inhibited or afraid of sex, but now I think it is wonderful and I embrace it more."

Barbara met Rick—"the right person," as she puts it—shortly after being pronounced cancer-free and turning 50. "It is funny, 50 was so liberating. I don't feel so locked into doing things a certain way. I've always been a controlling kind of person who wants things done the right way. If I'd see a typo on a handout that I was giving out I would be just so mad at myself. But I realized after I turned 50 and went through all that stuff with the cancer, it just doesn't matter so much. I was handing something out with a big typo on it and I went 'Phooey!' you know, it was like 'Who cares!' I am less hard on myself now. That is my style now, and this man is so incredibly creative and sees things in so many ways that things don't have to be perfect because there are so many ways to do them. His attitude has really helped me a lot."

Barbara's new perspective and the open communication she has with Rick have played themselves out to her great advantage in their sexual relationship. "It is just not as easy now to get fulfilled as it used to be, so you kind of go with the flow. I have a lot of trouble having orgasm. I don't know if that's from the chemotherapy or just my low libido, but sometimes I have to use a vibrator. Our sex is wonderful, but I don't orgasm (with intercourse). I go with the flow now; if my sexual desire is not fulfilled I don't feel badly about it. I'm not going to worry about it. Something will happen later. It didn't used to be like that. I used to feel so much more pressure."

We were quite impressed with Barbara's dramatic attitude shift and how it benefited her sexual life. She has been able to "go with the flow" and accept the new reality of her altered sexual responsiveness in spite of being confronted with the same pressures that our culture exerts on all older women.

As we address in Chapter 8, the quality of your relationship with your intimate partner can be a primary influence not only on your level of desire but on how you respond to physical illness or injury. With the assistance of a loving and flexible partner, adjusting to the consequences of illness or injury can yield huge rewards for a woman's sexual self-esteem. What happens, though, when it is the partner whose health is damaged?

When a Partner Is Ill

At 78, Lois was diagnosed with uterine cancer and a hysterectomy was required. "Just before that Tom developed Parkinson's and prostate cancer. After his operation he couldn't get an erection. It was a difficult time because he wanted to so badly, and he would work so hard at it. But it just became a painful process—he would try to stimulate me orally or manually and that would get me all steamed up all right, but then where do you go? And so I told him let's just stop because it is painful for both of us. With my hysterectomy my desire dropped and it has been easier to just close it off. Tom was out of commission too by that time, so it was just kind of a mutual thing. But we still hugged each other and you know we had some physical contact, but didn't have intercourse. He's not doing well, but I just hug him tight. He's a great husband. We had some fine times. I'm grateful."

Statistically, women do better health-wise than men as they get into their 70s and 80s. Among the women in our study, those with partners over 75 frequently referred to the fact that their partner's poor health had limited their sexual lives considerably. Nonetheless, we heard many descriptions of how these couples maintained physical and emotional intimacy by keeping in touch with each other.

Today Lois is 84. She lives in a small bungalow that her son built behind his home. This way she gets to see her grandkids regularly, and she isn't too far from the nursing home where Tom is living. Her husband of sixty-two years now requires more physical care than Lois is able to manage. Sex had been a vital part of their relationship. "When we were young it was the most normal thing. I just can't believe that there is anyone that doesn't have a sexual urge. For us it was just fun. I still would have strong urges even after menopause. I can remember we just had really fine times. But it really just came to a halt after his operation. That was quite a long time ago; in fact, I wouldn't know what to do sexually now it has been so long. I guess you just relax and go along with it."

Belinda, is a 64-year-old Bostonian now living in Georgia. The flame of desire has burned brightly throughout her 28-year marriage to David. They've weathered many storms together, and their relationship has been solid through it all. In the last four years, Belinda and David have faced a new challenge with his diagnosis of cancer. "This is," as she puts it, "a whole other tune to dance to. It has been so difficult for my husband and me to have intercourse since he's been on hormone suppression therapy for cancer. Once he couldn't become aroused without Viagra—and there were terrible side effects from that—I felt it wasn't worth it. I mean, putting him through that; he felt so bad because he couldn't satisfy me.

"It's been interesting for me: in the last few years my degree of desire has really declined. I think that's divine intervention so I won't become so frustrated. But I still have these waves, when I have an extreme amount of desire. I take care of them with fantasy. Sexual fantasy was very, very important to me during the years after I was divorced. I have to admit I am still surprised when these waves come to me where I have so much strong fantasy because I have so

Miss Bea

Eighty-year-old Miss Bea, the church organist, had never been married. She was much admired for her sweetness and kindness to all.

The pastor came to call on her one afternoon early in the spring, and she welcomed him into her Victorian parlor. She invited him to have a seat while she prepared a little tea. As he sat facing her old pump organ, the young minister noticed a cut glass bowl sitting on top of it, filled with water. In the water floated, of all things, a condom. Imagine his surprise and shock. Imagine his curiosity! Surely Miss Bea had flipped or something.

When she returned with tea and cookies, they began to chat. The pastor tried to stifle his curiosity about the bowl of water and its strange contents, but soon it got the better of him, and he could no longer resist. Pointing to the bowl, he asked, "Miss Bea, I wonder if you would tell me about this."

"Oh yes," she replied. "Isn't it just wonderful? I was walking downtown last fall and I found this little package on the ground. The directions said to put it on the organ, keep it wet, and it would prevent disease. And you know, I haven't had a cold all winter."

much desire. I thought that they would just go away, but they always surprise me when they come back."

Aside from fantasy, Belinda has another outlet for her sexual energy. "I sing in a really, really outstanding chorus. Music is very important to me and is a powerful emotional release." She is also able to see a lot of men in tuxedos: "We perform in black gowns and tuxedos. There is something extremely sexy about a man in a tuxedo. I don't know where it comes from, all I know is that when we are in our rehearsal room before a concert and 20 of the 40 people in that room are men in tuxedos...I just think that's pretty sexy." And on occasion, when Belinda and David are invited to a black-tie event, they look at each other in that old way and enjoy the tingle.

Belinda has found that coping with her husband's inability to perform sexually is taxing at times, but there is still a strong spark between them and she focuses on her gratitude and relief that he has survived his illness.

Other women have a different viewpoint. A number of women talked about how a debilitating illness in their partner can be a sad and frustrating experience. For example, Toni, a lively 65-year-old dance instructor, described her marriage this way: "My husband has lost interest in sex because he takes heart medication. I am resentful about this and it is not fair. He doesn't seem to care about my needs anymore and I really resent it."

> No intercourse in the last year. He had prostate cancer with radiation so no erection. Caring, kissing, hugging companionship is what we have now.
>
> —*Grace, 75, New Orleans, Louisiana*

And at 57, Jill, a registered nurse, is resigned: "My husband is diabetic and cannot keep an erection. We don't have sex. You'd think with my nursing background we could figure something out. But we haven't."

But Francis, who is 51, has found it possible to talk with her partner, and they are approaching the problem together: "I am desirous of my partner who has an illness that inhibits his sexuality and desire. I am frustrated at times, understanding at times. We are currently trying to redefine sex and work out new options."

Talking About the Effects of an Illness

How do you talk about your separate sexual needs when one of you has major health issues that interfere with sexual functioning? Certainly if you have fostered open communication about sexuality throughout your relationship, this is a much less daunting task. But for a huge proportion of couples, the first time they feel a need to talk about their sexual desires with each other is when one of them is confronted with a serious health crisis. This is one of the indirect ways in which changes in your or your partner's health can lead to a stronger connection between you. Facing an illness together can open the door to new levels of emotional intimacy.

Barbara, who met Rick after surviving two bouts of cancer, talked about how her partner's attitude helped her to be more self-accepting and to appreciate her sexual sensations. She was describing one way a supportive and caring mate can promote sexual balance in a health-challenged relationship. Francis and her partner have recognized that by "redefining sex" and considering options for sexual pleasure other than traditional intercourse, they are growing more intimate.

The basic guidelines that facilitate open communication about sexuality in general apply here in spades: remember that this isn't a topic you can cover in a single conversation; find opportunities to talk when you are both relaxed—and preferably not when you are in bed. Turn toward each other so you give your partner your full attention. Check out the suggestions at the end of Chapter 8 for more specifics.

It can also be very helpful to talk about your sexual desire with your women friends or with the people in your support group if you have one. There are also a number of resources that offer suggestions for dealing with specific illnesses that impact sexuality, and we have listed several at the end of this chapter.

Can Sexual Self-Esteem Survive a Serious Illness?

Regardless of whether you are currently partnered or not, facing a serious illness can change your self-perception and make you feel less sexually desirable. In much the same way that the predictable changes that occur in women's bodies as we age can cause damage to our sexual self-esteem, being ill or injured can put you at odds with our own body. You may feel that you aren't as self-reliant as you once were. If your image of yourself encompassed being a caretaker for others, it can be startling and disorienting to find yourself in need of care from others. Even though we all know laughter is healing, it may be hard to tune in to the optimistic, humorous side of yourself when you are scared and in pain. And if there are changes in your body's response to sensation as a result of medications or chemotherapy, as many of the women who have gone through cancer treatment described, your reliable source of pleasure from sexual stimulation may be missing.

> I'm surprised to find I have so little sexual desire. Could it be due to taking Premarin? Also, due to chronic pain and arthritis in my hip, limited range of motion restricts my ability to play and limits positions. I'm a person who likes variety, so perhaps the pain has depressed my desire. It surfaces in my dreams, so obviously I'm still capable of feeling arousal.
>
> —*Alice, 53, Portland, Maine*

How do women find their way back to positive sexual self-esteem when they have been dealt such a blow?

When we met Ursula, a 67-year-old bisexual, she was over-joyed to be in a settled and committed relationship with Darlene. But much of her energy was devoted to coping with physical pain. "It was 1993 or 1994 when I was first diagnosed with a repetitive stress injury. And then that morphed into fibromyalgia, which I ended up getting a doctor's diagnosis for, and then I was seeing an acupuncturist. He said, you know, we really should be looking at arthritis. So I got myself into the clinical trial, and luckily, I paid 'humma humma' to the right goddess and got on the Embrel side rather than the placebo side. I don't know where I would be right now if that hadn't happened. I don't know where Darlene and I would be. I sense that I would probably be in a nursing home because it was that bad.

"Because of having psoriatic arthritis and taking the Embrel, Darlene and I have not physically been able to be doing sexual acts per se. But Darlene and I are very loving towards each other and I just don't think at this stage in our lives we're missing anything. We've both 'been there done that.' And so we look at it in a different way now than we would have done earlier in our lives. We just recognize that this is what is happening in our lives right now and it will calm down when I have gotten a better handle on the psoriatic arthritis. The pain is being treated now with this medication, which in essence dampens down my auto-immune system—it's an immune depressor, but in its immune depressing it also cuts back the pain so that I actually have a life. It's amazing. It's magic."

Ursula has been able to come to terms with severe limitations on her sexual activity and drastic changes in the way her body feels and functions while remaining sexually alive. She makes conscious efforts to express her affection toward her partner and to continue to give voice to her own creativity.

Dawn was a high school teacher, married with two young

children, when she slipped on the stairs and ended up with a spinal cord injury. After a long rehab, she regained her mobility but was left with severe chronic pain. The only solution that was acceptable to her was having a morphine pump implanted in her body. At that point in her life, Dawn and her husband were having a lot of problems. "I didn't think about the fact that my sexual desire was shut off by the morphine pump because my husband and I didn't really want to have anything to do with each other sexually. And then he came out of the closet. I had been married twenty years, and I had no idea he was gay. But then so many things fell into place and I thought 'oh my God, how could I have been so stupid?' But it was kind of a relief to find out.

"It's amazing how a person can whittle your self-esteem down to nothing. I just thought I was a slug, so I just really never thought about sex much during our marriage. And then we divorced and I didn't think about it much afterwards because I had that pump which numbed me. I think I kind of redirected my sexual energy during that period. I'm an artist and I paint and I quilt and I threw myself into that. I was still teaching and I got my master's degree at that time. All of that helped me to build my self-esteem back up.

"But then, just this year, I told the doctor I wanted to go on a trial without the morphine. And, oh my God, my sensations are back! I didn't realize I was numb. It's like awakening from a sleep. I think it's wrong for doctors not to tell you about all the side effects."

Dawn fostered her self-esteem by channeling her energies into areas of creative and educational development. She lives alone and does not have a sexual partner, but she has embraced the return of sensual sensations and is delighted to find that she is still a sexual being. She continues to struggle with limited mobility and to be sidelined by pain frequently, but Dawn has found her way back to herself. Could she have gotten on this path to healing more easily if she had had more open channels of communication with her doctor? It's possible. If you are struggling with a physical condition that affects your sexuality, there are some things you can do to make your conversations with your health care provider more relevant to your needs.

Talking with Your Doctor

Dawn's comments about communication with her doctors were echoed by many women who had found it difficult to get straight, helpful information about how the medications they were taking or the illnesses they suffered were affecting their sexual lives. While many women say their physician is the person with whom they would be most likely to discuss sexual issues, a majority of post-menopausal women claim that their physician doesn't bring it up or does so only when the patient first raises the topic. In fact, less than half of older women patients report that their physicians ask them about sexual issues, according to a survey conducted in 2003 by the Association of Reproductive Health Professionals.

If you are coping with an illness that is affecting your sexual feelings, or if you and/or your partner are taking a new medication and you're not sure if there are sexual side effects, you need to have a conversation with your health-care provider.

Tips for getting the most out of your 15 minutes with your physician:

1. **Make a list of your questions ahead of time (and don't forget to bring it with you!).** Even those burning questions that prompted you to make the appointment in the first place tend to get forgotten without a note to jog your overloaded brain. List the most important ones first, so they'll be sure to get discussed.

2. **You can (and probably should) be the one to start the conversation.** Physicians have told us that they are unlikely to bring up this topic for fear of offending or embarrassing you.

3. **Don't wait till you're getting dressed to bring it up!** Tell your doctor early in the appointment that you have some questions about sexuality to discuss. You don't want the limited amount of time to get all taken up before you've had a chance to raise your concerns. Whether your doctor is a good listener or not, she or he will likely prefer to know what your concerns are up front rather than having to guess.

4. **Your annual exam is most often a longer appointment and is a good time to bring up sexual questions.** This is a complex topic and it's likely that you'll want more than 15 minutes to explore it. On the other hand, you don't want to wait a whole year for this conversation, so if your annual exam is a ways off, ask for a little extra time when you make your appointment.

5. **Don't be put off by jargon or big words or big egos.** Ask for further explanation. If you don't understand something, ask your doctor to tell you again. If you don't ask, your healthcare provider is likely to assume that you understood what was said. Once you have presented your concerns and your doctor has given you some information, summarize and repeat out loud what you heard to be sure you got it right. This gives the clinician an opportunity to clarify if you missed something.

6. **If your doctor prescribes any medication for you, ask about the possibility of sexual side effects.** It is amazing how many medications today can interfere with your sexual desire, arousal, or response; these include medications for hypertension, cancer treatment, diabetes, and depression, to name just a few.

7. **Consider taking notes or bringing a tape recorder to help you remember.** If you want to record what is being said, be sure to ask first! If you feel comfortable doing so, ask a friend or your spouse or partner to come with you. Two memories are better than one.

8. **Ask for written information.** Perhaps your doctor has a brochure or an audio or video tape. If not, ask where you can get more information.

9. **After the visit, review your notes to see if you have any further questions.** If you do, make another appointment or ask for a referral to a specialist or counselor.

10. **Be sure to follow through on suggestions your doctor gives you.**

11. **Be brave!**

Resources for Information About the Sexual Impact of Illness

National Association of Senior Friends: www.seniorfriends.org

The Arthritis Foundation: www.arthritis.org

The American Heart Association: www.Americanheart.org. The AHA publishes two pamphlets that are particularly helpful: "Sex After Stroke" and "Sex and Heart Disease."

Information on diabetes and sex: www.lifeclinic.com/focus/diabetes/sex.asp

Information on breast cancer and sex: www.breastcancer.org

Information on cancer in general and sex: www.cancer.org

Confronting changes in one's own health or the health of a partner is a hallmark of aging. Some of the most poignant questions women asked us in gatherings throughout the country had to do with how sickness or a chronic ailment would alter their sexual desire and sexual behavior. The more urgent, and yet unspoken, question was, "How do I maintain a positive sexual self-image in spite of illness or injury?" Although illness can be a blow to sexual self-confidence and drugs can dull responsiveness, there are many alternative paths to intimacy available to women. As the stories in this chapter demonstrate, effective communication between women and their partners as well as that between patients and their doctors is key to providing genuine support and understanding to a woman who is struggling with serious illness.

Truth #8

Women Over 50 Can Redefine Intimacy

What Older Women Want Out of Their Relationships...and How to Talk About It

Marlene glanced at the calendar as she finished up the breakfast dishes. "Valentine's Day, wow," she felt her stomach lurch. She'd met Brian thirty-seven years earlier on a brilliantly sunny February morning. They'd been invited to brunch at the home of mutual friends and ended up spending the whole day together walking and talking. The day had been so charged with sexual energy they couldn't help falling in lust with each other.

It was 1968; they were both in their 20s and swept up into the political climate of the time. They moved in together and battled over mundane stuff, patching up every fight with passionate sex. After a few years they had married. "To please our parents" was the explanation they'd voiced, but the idea of commitment and starting a family had appealed to both of them. Over the decades, they had faced their share of hard times. Brian struggled to get his career going while Marlene's success came quickly. This imbalance was tough and had forced them to learn new ways to be supportive of each other. Marlene was pregnant with their first child when her mother died. Left to cope with the world of parenthood without the benefit of her own mother's wisdom, Marlene had leaned heavily on Brian. After a few rough starts, he'd proven up to the task of father as well as husband. The years of parenting together had delighted and exhausted them. Over time, their relationship had fallen into a comfortable pattern that provided them both with the companionship and affection they needed.

But something had shifted in the last several years, and Marlene found herself dreading February—the month of romance—because it made the contrast so blatant. The distance between her and Brian had been growing gradually, and now she could no longer ignore it. He hardly ever enveloped her in his arms like he used to as she stood at the stove making dinner. They frequently went to bed at different times and rarely kissed good night. And sex? "When was the last time?" Marlene searched her memory. It had been long enough in the past that she wasn't sure, and she doubted that it would happen again any time soon.

She knew Brian wasn't as sexually driven as he used to be, no doubt about it. His erections weren't as reliable, but then, neither was her response. She couldn't have sex without using a lubricant anymore. It wasn't that she didn't find him sexy or didn't care for him anymore. She loved Brian deeply. "At this point in life maybe this is just what happens. What did I expect? We're both getting older. I haven't been sleeping so well myself with these hot flashes. And then there's the weight gain. Brian has never been judgmental about my body, but these days I can't be much of a turn-on to him when I can't stand to look at myself. Since he isn't as interested, maybe I should just let it go." But it wasn't the sex that she missed so much; she longed for their old intimacy.

Marlene realized that if she were feeling like this, Brian was probably unhappy, too. She had learned that the indirect approach was not a good idea with Brian—he never seemed to pick up on her studied, subtle messages. If she was angry with him she had to tell him so point blank or he'd just think she was in a bad mood. "Okay, I'll give it a try," she thought as she considered her dinner menu in honor of St. Valentine. When he came in the door, Marlene laid it out, "Brian, I want to talk. I miss you. Here it is Valentine's Day, and we haven't even hugged each other. I don't like what's been happening to us."

He sighed, "I'm sorry, honey, I just feel so old lately—it's getting me down I think. I don't feel much like having sex."

"That's not what I mean, Brian. We can be close and not have sex." Marlene realized that they hadn't talked about their relationship in a very long time. "Here, Brian, have a glass of wine. I'd like us to toast to love and romance. Let me tell you what's been going on with me, and I want to hear about what's happening for you. Getting older is much more complicated than I thought it would be." Marlene and Brian began facing aging together. It was a process that involved exploring what they wanted their relationship to feel like for the next 25 years and, ultimately, redefining intimacy for themselves.

Reframing Notions of Intimacy

Intimacy and *sex* are not interchangeable terms, but we tend to use them that way. In general, for men intimacy is a metaphor for the sex act; for women, when they engage in the sex act, they are often looking for emotional intimacy. Sexual desire comes in waves for everyone, even for the most passionate of couples, but real intimacy is a deeper, more lasting bond. Women in our study made the point repeatedly: the qualities of an intimate relationship that hold the most meaning have more to do with emotional understanding than simply with physical appreciation of one another.

When women talk about wanting men to be more intimate,

what they generally mean is that they want men to share their emotional experiences more openly. This can be a very difficult task for men who have been raised to ignore their feelings or at least to keep them hidden. Beverly, 82, put it this way: "So many men are puzzled by women because they are not in touch with their own feelings...When a man can just let himself enjoy women as other human beings...in other words, it's a human issue."

What is certain is that intimacy and healthy relationships go together like a horse and carriage—you can't have one without the other. When faced with the possibility of change—particularly in an arena like aging or sexual desire—even the most confident person can feel vulnerable. Couples tend to retreat into silence or make assumptions about each other. In newer relationships in which the patterns aren't as set, couples may avoid such a sensitive subject and instead make educated guesses about how they think their partner feels. Even a smooth, comfortable, well-oiled relationship can easily turn into a tangle of misunderstandings. Rather than building roads to greater intimacy together, older couples can drive themselves miles apart.

Just as women find it beneficial to take stock of their personal sexual health once they've celebrated their 50th birthdays, their relationships also need nurturing attention. A multitude of women told us the connection between the health of their intimate relationships and their personal sexuality is mighty strong.

Intimacy, Sexual Desire, and the Love Relationship

Midori and Craig

Born in Japan, Midori came to this country as a young wife. She struggled with her "confusion about love" as she puts it, from the very beginning. Now at 62, her understanding of intimacy is a very soulful concept that goes far beyond the physical. Midori's marriage to Kei was arranged by their families. He was many years older than she, and her desires were not considered at the time, even by her. As Midori describes it, "I married the man my parents chose and I was content with him, but there was no love." They moved to the United States when Midori was barely 21 and had only a rudimentary knowledge of English. She was totally dependent on Kei for managing in the new world they had entered. Bound by tradition, their relationship was polite. Midori stayed close to home, working diligently on her language skills. Then the birth of her child opened a door for her. At the hospital where her baby was born, she joined a support group for young mothers that gave her the opportunity to meet others struggling to figure out what to do with upside-down schedules, screaming babies, and low sexual desire. Gradually, she made some friends and began to find her way in an unfamiliar culture. The more independent she became, the less connected to Kei she felt.

By the time their son was a teenager, Midori acknowledged that she had become quite Americanized. "I attended college, met similarly minded women, and learned to speak out about the meaning of love, which markedly altered my relationship with Kei. Eventually, I left Kei and moved into my own apartment." After completing college and finding a job that encouraged the development of her creative talents, Midori's self-confidence flowered. "Something started changing after I was 40 or so. I became aware of my shortening life span and I got more brave. I began to encounter relationships with men more boldly and became a more active participant."

> As I struggle with aging body image, being desired (both physically and emotionally) is more important. Sex is slower, deeper, more bonding.
>
> —*Sharon, 58, Orlando, Florida*

It was in this newly blossoming persona that Midori met Craig. Theirs is a relationship she wants to nurture for a long time. "We both feel that the spiritual aspect of our union is very important; and we are good friends. I know now that relationships ebb and flow. For me, developing trust and an open heart is the goal. For much of my marriage, sex was only a duty that I, as a good wife, had to provide. Kei and I never talked about sex and intimacy and what it all means. In my relationship with Craig I have learned to express my needs and to listen to what he is feeling. We have a kind of intimacy that I never realized was possible. It is something that goes way beyond the physical. If I had not been willing to be bold I don't know if I would have ever found what Craig and I have. Now that we are getting older, I am so very grateful that we have the kind of bond that we do. We can talk, we can fight, we can sit in church and hold hands."

How many older women would claim that they had found the model relationship Midori has discovered? In a somewhat naïve effort to quantify this, we included a forced choice question on our survey. We asked women, "How do you feel about your partner as a lover?" We offered them the following options: passionate, satisfied, uninterested, or resentful. Most of the women who answered this question were either passionate or satisfied, but it was also clear that such simplified answers missed the point for an awful lot of

An Unspoken Truth

"How do you feel about your partner as a lover?"

A. Passionate about partner as lover — 22%

B. Satisfied with partner as lover — 35%

C. Uninterested in partner as lover — 7%

D. Resentful toward partner as lover — 3%

E. Don't currently have a sexual partner — 22%

F. No answer — 11%

women. This question didn't make sense to them because their understanding of intimacy was much more complex than what these four options described.

Elaine and Daniel

One might expect that, like many of the long-married respondents in our study, 58-year-old Elaine would have described herself as being satisfied with her former husband as a lover. But sexual performance or frequency of sex isn't what determines the quality of the love relationship. These days Elaine lives in a condo in Phoenix. Four years ago she left her husband of 25 years and moved from the wet Northwest to the sun. In the early years of their marriage, Elaine and Daniel had enjoyed a passionate, satisfying sexual life together. After their kids were born, life took on that typical hectic pace that leaves little time for romantic attention. That was okay with Elaine—after all, she told us, "I was exhausted most of the time anyway." But once their children were older and needed less, Elaine wanted more emotional closeness with Daniel. He didn't seem to understand what she wanted. Elaine said she felt discarded and unappealing because Daniel didn't crave physical closeness either and would withdraw from her rather than talk about what was troubling him. Resentment set in, eventually leading to divorce. "It took me a long time to realize I didn't want to live like that. I felt I really didn't have self-esteem, I wasn't feeling like I had any desire, any libido, or that I was desirable for anyone else."

As in Elaine and Daniel's situation, if older couples don't communicate their needs, especially when they have a history of expressing their affection through sex, the disparate changes in their sexual desire can lead to serious hurt. Communication, as we all know, is a two-way street. Women and men are equally responsible for expressing their needs. Poor communication patterns established early in a relationship make it even more difficult to revitalize a discordant relationship.

Linda and Mike

Linda was born and raised in the same small town in Iowa where she lives today. Her image of a happy marriage came more from what she saw on TV than from real life.

During her self-conscious high school years, Linda's first boy-friend was a young football player named George. "Boy, did he arouse my passion! We were both 'steeped in Lutheran guilt,' so our desire led only to kissing and hugging." When Linda was a junior in college, she began dating Mike, who was also from her hometown. "We had common backgrounds and felt comfortable with each other right away. I didn't feel the level of passion I felt for George, but it really didn't concern me at the time.

She married Mike at age 23, but today, some 30 years later, she looks back on her decision with regret. "I can vividly remember this...we were married in December. We graduated from college and left on the 22nd, and got married on the 28th. There was snow and it was cold. I was walking from my parents' home hearing the crunching of the snow, going to the car, driving to the church, thinking 'Linda, you shouldn't be doing this, but it's too late now. You have to.'"

Over the ensuing 20 years, Linda and Mike had three children and lived a conservative life in that small midwestern city. Her sexual passion never got ignited during those years, but she was busy and she continued to perform in her compliant manner. "What bothered me was his expectation that because we were married he had the right to have intercourse with me, whether I was ready or wanting to right then or not." She didn't describe Mike as abusive but used words like *controlling* and *demanding*. "In many

> Passion about my lover is not necessarily related to the frequency of our sex.
>
> —*Mary, 62, Corpus Christi, Texas*

ways, the relationship was all about him. I never felt that he understood me or how I felt."

Linda pursued her professional career, slowly gaining more responsibility and authority. Then, in her 40s, she met someone. The chemistry, as she calls it, was electric. "It made me feel alive again. Meeting someone else made me feel like I wanted to have a sexual relationship. I was surprised that anybody would be interested in me." It was a passionate connection that lasted three years; through it Linda learned a lot about what an intimate relationship could feel like. By the time she was 52, she had had a second sexual relationship outside of her marriage.

Today Linda is still married to Mike. They have a friendship of sorts but live very separate lives. She doesn't feel any desire for him, and they haven't had sex for three years. "We have come to this not without some pain and arguments and so forth, but we have come to a kind of agreement that this is how it is. I have been more accepting of that than he has, but there isn't the tension any more between us. It is easier to be friends and be nice to each other. We actually enjoy doing a few things together once in a while."

At least for the time being, Linda has chosen to remain celibate within her marriage. She continues to have dreams of sexual intimacy, though: "I would like my sexual desire to be high, and I would love to have a close intimate, meaningful, passionate relationship with someone I really truly cared about. I haven't given up on that dream yet. I do think it is still possible, even when you are 85 or 90 years old."

> To me sexual desire is wanting to be with somebody. The reason that I originally became involved sexually with my partner was that I knew that I would never get to really know her well till I was more intimate with her.
>
> —*Alice, 67-year-old lesbian, Oklahoma*

Desire Intertwined

As in Linda's case, women in our study often talked about how intricately interwoven their own sexual desire was with that of their partner and how his, or sometimes her, level of sexual interest stimulated their own sexual feelings. For Judy, it took a long time to find a relationship where this worked in her favor, but at 60 she feels she's found it. "I met my current husband just after my 50th birthday. I have always had strong sexual desire, but because of him and his caring about me in all parts of our life together, my satisfaction and desire are greater than ever. He is a cuddler and a toucher, as well as being a skilled lover."

Sometimes, though, the physical changes that accompany aging can have a different kind of impact on this interaction between partners and their levels of desire. Some women still want to have sex with their partner but feel thwarted because he is unable to achieve an erection. In some cases, when a partner has erectile difficulties, he turns away from his wife or lover, completely losing sight of her needs and only focusing on his. Inez from Dallas described how her husband couldn't even bring himself to say the word *impotent* for months.

> It is discouraging that my spouse seems less interested in sex than he used to be.
>
> —*Lotty, 66, Arkansas*

"Perhaps he couldn't pronounce the word, or perhaps he was too embarrassed to admit what was going on." Finally, he agreed to see a physician who gave him a prescription for Viagra. When that didn't work, he simply gave up. "My husband has been absolutely inconsiderate when it comes to my sexual needs. I guess he thinks that if he can't have an erection, then I can't get turned on. He won't even talk about it. I'm frustrated and frankly, pretty mad at him."

Gina has taken a different tack. She's titrated her own desire to match her husband's lowered sexual appetite. She told us, "When one's partner has a reduced libido, one adapts one's own desires accordingly." When there is a significant disparity in the level of sexual desire within a couple, it can be a daunting task to find a path to intimacy.

Anna and Bob

We first met Anna in Chapter 7, when she described how she copes with her diabetes, but her story really begins in 1942. In her late teens, she started her career as an Army nurse. "I was 18 and away from home for the first time when I was drawn to Bob. We'd both been raised in Texas and provided a little bit of 'home' for each other in the midst of the chaos of war. Not only that, but I felt a lust for Bob that made me forget all the other guys around." They married, but the pressures on the twosome were intense. As a military couple, they had little control over their own lives. They managed to stay together long enough to have a daughter, Mae. But the circumstances were tough, and their sexual passion fizzled under the weight of parental responsibility. Soon both Anna and Bob sought escape. They agreed to divorce when Mae was 5 years old.

The challenge of raising Mae on her own drove Anna to look for more dependability in the men she dated. Anna eventually found Charlie, a stable, sweet man and a loving father. "I felt relaxed with him and trusted his kind heart. Our marriage looked and felt very different from my first one. We raised Mae together, grew older, and felt quite settled.

"But you know, my sexual desire was always at a high pitch. Over the years I came to recognize that Charlie was not as sexually oriented as me. In time we were able to come to an accommodation that I thought satisfied us both." But when Charlie retired, his interest in sex dropped dramatically. At first, Anna felt hurt and rejected.

"I still desired him; I still felt young and vital." In spite of her efforts to reawaken their sexual life, Charlie made it clear that, though he loved her, sex was over for him. Anna tried to accept this, but it was a difficult struggle for her. Eventually, Charlie withdrew emotionally as well and was unwilling to talk with Anna about her needs. "As I got older I found that I could handle the lack of sex much more easily than the lack of emotional connection. He may have been depressed; he just wouldn't talk. I felt lonely."

When she was 69 years old, her daughter turned 50. "Mae threw a big party for herself, inviting all the important people in her life, including Charlie and me. Charlie opted not to take the trip to Texas. He said it was too far and that he and Mae hadn't been that close." Anna, however, wouldn't have missed it for the world. And neither would Bob, Mae's biological father.

At the party, Anna and Bob found themselves alone together for the first time in 45 years. They quickly discovered that the spark was still very much alive between them. Here was her soul mate, Anna realized. And now that they were both older, they had a deeper appreciation for the emotional intimacy Anna had been hungering for. While she still felt great fondness for Charlie, Anna needed more than he could give. It was not an easy decision for her. She talked with Charlie and was surprised to learn that he could understand her need for what Bob offered. He knew that the kind of closeness Anna wanted was uncomfortable for him. Since their divorce, Anna and Charlie have remained friends. But it is with Bob

> I would say probably when I hit my mid-50s or so my sexual desire seemed to slow down. It wasn't as important; I didn't think about sex as much. But I think in general, it's not the sex so much, but the desire to be with someone, to have that caressing and that cuddling rather than the act of sex itself, although that's still important, but not as important.
>
> —*Corky, 61-year-old, New York*

that Anna feels most completely at home. Age and illness have limited their physical intimacy; they have sex infrequently but nurture their emotional and mental connection with long talks and shared dreams. "I know he loves me—he tells me all the time. I feel so lucky because I know what it's like to live without that."

Less Can Be More

Many women who have been in long-term relationships echoed Anna's experience with Bob when they spoke to us about how things had changed for them sexually. They may not engage in the sex act itself as often as they did when they were younger, but when they do, the experience is more fulfilling, more intimate than it used to be. Patricia, a retired cook who lives with her husband in south Florida, wrote, "The older I get, the more enjoyable it is to have an intimate relationship with my partner, but it doesn't always involve a sexual encounter. The goal is intimacy, sharing of the inner self as well as the body. My partner enjoys the sex more than I do, but we both enjoy the closeness and that is the most important part."

Regardless of sexual orientation, the connection between sexual desire, sexual self-esteem, and the quality of one's intimate relationship is indisputable. Molly is 59 and divorced; she is now in a committed relationship with another woman: "My sexual desire is greater than it used to be but it's because I'm in the right relationship. Maybe in my marriages, I had a desire to have sex, but I just didn't have much of a desire to have sex with my former husbands. I want to emphasize my strong belief that a healthy relationship is key to sexual desire. Really, though, my sexual desire could be strong, but if the relationship is not meeting my needs, then why have sex? I think that reading a book called *In the Meantime* by Iyanla Vanzant puts what I'm trying to say in perspective. She talks about relationship as levels of a house. The first relationship feels as though you're in the basement. Then, you go to the next relationship and you're in a different room, on a different level. Now, I'm all the way in the penthouse!"

Another point of view was offered by Melinda, a woman whose dramatic beauty draws attention whenever she enters a room. A 55-year-old Native American living near the Rocky Mountains, she and her third husband, Don, have been married for 16 years. "I believe in letting nature take its course, and there comes a time when, as we pass the age of child rearing, the desire is not as strong. There are times when I feel an urge to have sex with my husband—for whatever reason, there's this 'ping,' and I am more attracted to him sometimes. I'm just not as passionate about my husband as I once was." Melinda mentioned that she's asked Don, "Are you okay with our sex life the way it is? Are we having sex enough, does it feel like it's enough, is it fun enough?" And Don's response? "Yes, I'm happy with it." She went on, "So, sometimes we have sex once a month or once every two months, and on rare occasions, twice in a week. And we enjoy each other, regardless of the frequency of our love-making."

Those couples, like Melinda and Don, who understand that aging inevitably brings change and that intimacy can grow even if sexual interactions diminish, can work together to deepen their connection. But it can be a difficult task. With all the sexual self-esteem issues older women are contending with, they are often full of doubt about whether they are desirable anymore. A mate who is willing to say out loud, "You're beautiful" or "I love you," is taking a huge step toward fostering intimacy. But it goes beyond physical attractiveness—respect remains an essential component of a passionate relationship. Valuing each other as whole people means honoring your different life experiences, listening attentively, and expressing your appreciation for each other. As Patsy, a 55-year-old defense contractor from Norfolk, Virginia, told us, "It helps if you have a husband or a partner who always likes you just the way you are: you don't have to be anything else, you don't have to be 25 pounds lighter."

For many women, being past the childbearing years opens the door to an exciting and stimulating time when they feel a burst of energy and motivation to try new things. The man who can see and appreciate a woman as a whole person understands how important her creativity is to her sense of self. An independent, confident, and competent woman has much to give to a relationship if her partner is supportive. This is the true meaning of partnership—a relationship in which both parties feel fully appreciated and encouraged to develop their unique talents and skills.

Valerie and Sam

When Valerie's first marriage ended, she had "a little bit of the savings" and a lot of self-doubt. "I had a bad case of down-on-myself blues." She was young (22), and the dream of a white-picket family she had harbored since her childhood was shattered. "That's when I started to grow up. I had to find my way. My parents weren't able to support me financially, but they were glad I was out of that marriage."

She worked various low-paying jobs until she found a way to attend college. Eventually, she earned a master's degree. Valerie's interests were in the political arena, and she found that she had a talent for persuading people to see her point of view. "It's a heady feeling to be part of making a change in the world. I loved my work."

"I lived alone for a long time and I learned to appreciate it. It was twenty-seven years between my marriages. By the time I found Sam I was a very independent career woman with some power in my field." Sam had left a long-term marriage and was bruised and battered by years of conflict with his former wife. "It took us both a long time to decide to trust and open up to each other. He is a good man who had a lot of guilt about his divorce and I was used to being alone. We were really tentative with each other. I remember thinking, do I need this? But, you know, I guess I must have."

After getting to know each other well over a couple of busy years, Valerie and Sam decided to marry. He has three grown children who took a while to warm up to Valerie, adding stress she had not expected. The first few years of their marriage were focused on adjusting to each other's rhythms and finding ways to continue to carve out romantic time together. Then a new challenge presented itself when Sam developed cancer. "It was a scary time. I had to learn a lot really quickly. He was so sick and needed care, so I quit my job and did it. I was surprised to find that I didn't resent it, you know. He is such a considerate guy—even when he was so sick, he wanted to hear about me and he hated that I couldn't keep working. But he recovered, thank God, and the whole thing had a big impact on me.

"Amazingly, I didn't want to return to my job. Once I got off the fast track, I loved it. I'd never had a chance to indulge in my other interests much. Sam went back to work. He still needs that—it's his anchor and he gets so much satisfaction from it. But he has encouraged me to do what I want. I really love him for that. He misses me when I go off on a trip without him—and I do—but I know that he appreciates me—all of me, so when I come home he just wants to hear about what I did and learned." Valerie certainly sounds pretty happy, and the support she gets from Sam is feeding that joy and the solid intimate connection between them.

Finding Intimacy Regardless of Marital Status

According to the Social Security Administration, a girl born today can expect to live to be almost 79; a boy to about 74—a difference of about five years. As we age, though, gender differences in life expectancy decrease. A 50-year-old woman can expect to live to be

82, and a 50-year-old man can expect to live to be 78—a difference of only 4 years. But while men may be catching up to the life expectancy of women, it still leaves plenty of older women whose husbands have passed on. According to data generated by the U.S. Administration on Aging, in 2003 there were four times as many widows over the age of 65 as widowers. Approximately 11 percent of the women who participated

Marital Status of U.S. Women 45 Years and Older

Now married:	58.9%
Never married:	5.8%
Widowed:	21.9%
Divorced:	13.4%

Source: U.S. Census, 2000

in our study were widows. For many of them, the topic of sexual desire was ancient history that they had buried with their spouses. One 70-year-old widow in Spokane, Washington, said "After my husband died I forgot about sex." But it isn't just a memory issue. As 83-year-old Dixie, who lost her husband 15 years ago, describes it, "Sexual desire doesn't go away. It's the arousal from the opposite sex one needs. If there are no men in your life, then the arousal diminishes."

But what happens to that need for intimacy, for closeness and connection with another who knows you well? Certainly that doesn't disappear. Older women often meet a lot of their need for connection through their relationships with other women. Girlfriends, whether they chose to explore a sexual relationship as some of the women in Chapter 6 have or not, are an important source of intimacy for each other. And this fact is borne out by recent research findings. *The Seattle Times* (June 15, 2005) quotes Beverly Fehr of the University of Winnipeg in Manitoba, author of a scholarly study of friends titled "Friendship Processes." According to Fehr, "When a romantic relationship ends, a woman still has other sources of intimacy—her friends—and that provides her with another source of support." The *Times* article goes on to report that "at least 22 studies have shown that having social support decreases the heart-racing, blood pressure boosting responses that humans and other social animals have to stress and the hormones it sends surging."

As Trudy, a 70-year-old retired veterinary tech, said, "I have wonderful friends. Most of us are widows now—we've known each other for years. I don't know what I'd do without them. They are my support, my companions. We have so much fun together. And I can talk to them about anything!" Trudy moved from the home where she raised her four children to a condo in the building next door to where her two best friends live. They "spill the beans" with each other regularly.

Other nonsexual relationships in women's lives can provide the kind of intense emotional connection that fulfills the need for intimacy. Kay is a divorced, 55-year-old grandmother who lives alone in a house with two comfortable guest rooms and a big, warm four-poster bed that just invites snuggling. "One of the ways that I really get sensual pleasure in my life is through my grandchildren. For me it's not about sex, it's about fully being with someone. When Mary Kate [her 4-year-old granddaughter] and I are together, she sleeps with me and we wake up in the morning and we cuddle and tell stories, and it's just so sweet. And obviously there are plenty of pieces missing since she is a child and she is my granddaughter, but it's hard to separate it and put it in boxes. To me it's all part of sensuality and intimacy."

We also heard from a number of widows whose intimacy needs were so fulfilled by their marriage that they are like the 74-year-old woman who described her status on the back of her survey as "a widow, not looking."

At 58, Indira may typify this kind of widow. Her husband died when she was in her 40s. She still cherishes the memory of their sexual life. She told us, "I am still so hooked into the wonderful relationship I had with my husband that unless I found someone who I felt was equally a partner I probably wouldn't try to engage in a long-term relationship. There are so few men around my age that don't have a whole bunch of other stuff hanging on them that it's not worth the investment. I'm not interested in being anybody's other woman. And the type of man I'd choose to be involved with would be a professional person who at least had some interests related to my interests—art, the opera, and the symphony—things that I really enjoy. And to be in a relationship, I'd have to find something beyond those. Someone who also has some basic values and beliefs I share. And so I'm not putting out the energy to find someone because I was so content with what I had. I don't see that that is going to change. Maybe someone will walk up and I'll say 'Wow, there he is' but it hasn't happened yet."

Though it is working for Indira, few unpartnered women in their 50s and 60s would choose to live through old age alone. Some may engage in long-distance relationships, seeing their boyfriend every few months. For economic and family reasons, others may decide to stay single but have a special person in their lives. Others may remarry. Many may have limited options when it comes to responding to the physical side of sexual aging but want to nurture mature relationships to maintain and create the kind of intimacy and connection that brings joy and comfort. Others satisfy their need for emotional and mental connections through friendships and interaction with their offspring.

Finding the Intimacy You Desire

As the different life stories in this chapter demonstrate, intimacy is not a static, one-dimensional experience. What you are expecting with regard to intimacy in your relationship can determine what actually happens for you. And it is quite possible that your expectations for intimacy may not be the same as your partner's. These are realities that apply to all kinds of relationships, whether you're sharing your life with a man or a woman, whether you are even part of a couple or living on your own. If you believe that the longer you have known each other, the less you need to talk because you understand each other by now—you're likely to be in for some unpleasant surprises with the kinds of changes aging brings.

If you believe that now that you're this old, much of the business of life has calmed down and there is time for you to enjoy each other—you may be setting yourself up for big disappointment if you don't share that expectation with your partner. And if you are in a sexual relationship and either one of you expects that once you're this age sex is no longer important, that can be a self-fulfilling prophecy—even though your partner may not share that expectation with you. So finding ways to share your expectations is a major step toward reviving intimacy in relationships of all kinds. As a start it is always helpful to examine your own attitudes.

An Unspoken Truth for Men: Get Real!

It's not uncommon for guys to take trophy wives, "trading in" their long-time spouse for a younger, sleeker model. Women as "eye candy" remain valuable commodities. But men who buy into a skewed, unrealistic view of sex are being disrespectful and undignified. Martina, who has just turned 50, said, "Will you just ask these men to please grow up! My body isn't want it used to be, and neither is my husband's. And I do resent it when he keeps ogling younger women with great bodies—and sometimes turns to a XXX-rated Internet site. It really makes me squirm."

Defining Intimacy

Ask yourself the following questions:

1. What does the word *intimacy* mean to me?

2. What expectations do I have for how intimate connection can flourish?

3. What things do I do to foster intimacy?

4. What other things could I do that would improve intimacy in the future?

Your reactions to these questions can be the impetus to get you to reevaluate what's happening in your cherished relationships. You can talk to your children and your nieces and nephews about the importance of your relationship. Let your friends know how much they mean to you. If you're partnered, consider changing the relationship dynamics by asking them to answer the questions. It can be very enlightening to discuss these questions together.

Five Keys to Intimacy for Older Couples

If you are partnered and stumped about exactly how to proceed, here are some specifics you might find helpful. These are a distillation of suggestions and ideas we received from numerous women about what they felt were the building blocks of an honestly intimate relationship. We urge you to think about these ideas and talk about them with your partners, your friends, your intimates.

1. Tune in.

What women told us over and over is that they felt closest to their partners, more sexually interested, more intimately connected when their partners paid attention to them. Luella, a 52-year-old, twice-divorced real estate agent in South Carolina, said, "A man has to be able to listen to a woman about what she likes and what she doesn't like and what turns her on and what makes her feel good. Men need to learn to think like that." And of course, this works both ways. Ask yourself: *What are the things that my partner currently does that show me he is fostering intimacy? How do I do the same for him?* For instance, we all appreciate being listened to—how do you know when he is tuned in to you? In the parlance of couples therapy, "active listening skills" are helpful: turning toward your partner when he is talking to you, paraphrasing what you heard him say, asking clarifying questions, and making sure your body language matches your words are all important elements.

2. Talk.

This certainly isn't news but bears repeating. Communication never goes out of style. No matter how old you are or how long you've been together—in fact, the longer you've been together the easier it is to forget this—no one can read another's mind. As modern humans, we look for shortcuts. Making assumptions is a kind of emotional communication shortcut that often leads us in the wrong direction. Even if your hypothesis is correct, you're going to improve your relationship by checking to be sure. The power of this suggestion is illustrated

> If you can get only one line into their heads, tell them to pay attention.
>
> —*Annette, 64, Flagstaff, Arizona*

by Paula's situation. She has remained with her husband of 35 years but has found greater intimacy with men outside her marriage: "My husband never asked me 'What do you want? What do you need?' He thought he knew, but he is so wrong." Perhaps if she and her husband had found a way to foster their bond through communication when they were at an earlier stage in their relationship, the feelings of futility and resignation she's experiencing now might have been avoided. It's hard to talk about your troubles if you don't know where to start.

If you have decided to take a risk and plunge into a conversation about your changing sexuality, you may be wondering just how to begin. Of course, you will structure the dialogue to meet your own needs and style, but Elizabeth's approach may serve as a useful example. She, like Marlene whose story began this chapter, had been worried about some changes in her relationship with her

An Unspoken Truth for Men: Get Clean!

Men may have figured out that a clean and healthy appearance is a major requirement when they want to make a good impression, but apparently a lot of guys don't realize how important cleanliness is when it comes to intimate relationships. So many women mentioned men's hygiene that we concluded there must be a lot of men out there who either don't know or don't pay attention to some of the basics, e.g., using deodorant, showering daily, and cleaning their fingernails. How wrong they are! As Vicky says, "Overbearing cologne doesn't equate to strength. I admire men who have strength of character, determination, focus, and that kind of thing. Dumping on the aftershave does not do a thing except turn me off."

husband. They had not done a lot of talking about their sexual relationship over the years of their marriage, so this was new for her. After attending one of our house gatherings, she called to say that she had broken the ice with Gary by telling him: "Honey, I don't know if you've noticed, but sexually things are feeling different for me lately. I know much of the change has to do with getting older. We've never been 60 before, and we have no experience with what might happen for us sexually in the next five or ten years. I've imagined that we'd still be having sex right up till we couldn't move anymore. I wonder if that's your expectation too. I'd like to know what's happening for you, and I'd like to tell you what's going on with me."

We can't say if it's easier to get the conversation started when you've been partnered for a long time or if you're in a newer liaison. Lisa, who is 72 and divorced, told us how she initiated a talk with her "special person." She has been seeing Ron for several years, but they haven't had much conversation about what kind of intimacy they want as they move forward. This has been hard for Lisa because she cares a lot about Ron and isn't sure that they are on the same page about the future. She started with the topic of sex (brave Lisa!), and the conversation moved on from there to encompass much more. Here's how she began: "I've been thinking about my expectations. I was always told that people didn't have sex after a while, but I don't want that to happen to us. What about you? What do you expect as we grow older?"

3. Touch.

It's amazing how easy this is to mess up. We all crave physical touch—no, we're not talking about sex here, we're talking about touching. As one woman in her 80s said: "The touch of a hand when we're walking, the lock of hair kindly brushed back." The expression "keep in touch" is more meaningful in this content than in any other—you just have to take it literally. One of the significant factors that separates happy, satisfied couples from those who are not is that the first group touches more often during the day—not just in bed. A hug, a hand on a shoulder, a close snuggle on the couch . . . these things keep the intimate connection alive.

4. Take time and be open to change.

The changes that aging brings can become big issues, not just for couples who have been together a long time, but also for newer relationships. If we cling to intimacy patterns that may have worked for us in the past, it's kind of like trying to hold back the tide. It just can't be done. As we age, all the aches and pains and physiological changes are challenges to our emotional flexibility and creativity. But the general slowing that accompanies growing older can be a distinct advantage—giving us time to savor close contact. We heard from many women in this chapter about the joys of holding hands and leisurely cuddles. Valerie's husband Sam was slowed by his cancer, and their sexual connection changed dramatically. "I have learned something very important," says Valerie. "I find kissing a very, very fulfilling experience—it is very fulfilling even if we don't have sex. There's more to it, we feel very close when we take time to kiss."

> Slower and gentler gives my man lots of points.
> —*Susie, 73, Tallahassee, Florida*

5. Laugh together.

Humor is a powerful love potion. As Megan, a 54-year-old bank teller from Roseburg, Oregon, told us, "As I get older, it's not appearance

Sunday Morning Sex

On hearing that her elderly grandfather had just passed away, Susan went straight to her grandparent's house to visit her 95-year-old grandmother and comfort her. When she asked how her grandfather had died, her grandmother replied, "He had a heart attack while we were making love on Sunday morning."

Horrified, Susan told her grandmother that two people nearly 100 years old having sex would surely be asking for trouble. "Oh no, my dear," replied Granny. "Many years ago, realizing our advanced age, we figured out the best time to do it was when the church bells would start to ring. It was just the right rhythm. Nice and slow and even. Nothing too strenuous, simply in on the ding, and out on the dong." She paused, wiped away a tear, and then continued, "And if that damned ice cream truck hadn't come along, he'd still be alive today."

that matters nearly so much. I look for a sense of humor, the ability to laugh." There's plenty of evidence that laughter is truly the best medicine for healing. We say it is also a great way to juice up your passion. Sure, laughing may make some women "leak," but the potential benefits are pretty profound. Even when things seem to be at a low point, we can enjoy the inherent humor in a situation. As countless women told us, a man who makes them laugh is a real turn-on.

One word of caution: if your idea of a good joke is one that demeans women or men, or if your humor and your partner's are mismatched, be careful. It can be a turn-off, as Alexandra told us, "A man being silly or cute or funny (he believes) at a crucial moment of lovemaking is a turn-off. Humor is wonderful at the right moments, but not at a tender moment."

Our most intimate relationships are the stage where the drama of aging is played out in Technicolor and vivid detail. Graying hair, thickening waistlines, and wider feet are visual reminders that we're no longer spring chickens. We witness our partner's transformations through our own filters, and hope to heaven that the changes our own bodies are going through are being regarded through his or her most loving lens.

Concurrently, the quality of our intimate interactions is evolving, even though this shift may be less visible to us. We may feel vulnerable, lonely, afraid—those old feelings we thought we'd put to rest about the time we graduated into adulthood—may once again be front and center. Our sexual self-confidence is at risk of sinking under the weight of physical and emotional needs we're experiencing.

Without directly addressing how aging is altering your intimate relationship, you can easily drift, as Marlene and Brian were, into a less-connected, but still companionable old age. For some couples, that can be a welcome relief. Many couples will want to acknowledge the shifts as Melinda did when she asked Don, "Are you happy with our sex life?" It takes courage and a willingness to abandon old patterns and to examine your relationship needs in light of your age. But if your vision of the future includes a new kind of passion and connection, you can redefine intimacy for yourselves.

Colette's story is a wonderful model for us all. Her tale came to us via the post; at 85, her flowing longhand was a pleasure to read. Her relationship with Roger began at their 65th high school reunion, when they reconnected after decades of no contact. Theirs is a long-distance relationship that has beaten the odds, and the kind of intimacy they share is nothing like what Colette had ever imagined. "I thought that at this age, if I found a man, it would be holding hands and kissing on the cheek, but this is like someone casually throwing a firecracker into a dump full of pyrotechnics. He lives 600 miles away, but we've been able to see each other often. We enjoy each other fully and are grateful for what we have, although at times, I'm not certain of what it is we have. It doesn't fit a pattern and often appears a patch-work affair, but it's a warm, tempestuous coming-together of two people who have found an unexpected treasure. We hold it tightly and sometimes lightly, but find special pleasure in each other."

Truth #9

It's Never Too Late to Celebrate Your Sexuality

Leaving Your Legacy

Luxuriating in the calm of her home and the softness of her bed, Sonia lay unmoving for a moment, listening to the doves cooing in the dark shelter of her balcony. There was no need to jump up; the alarm wasn't even set. She had the whole day ahead of her. It almost felt as if she were getting away with something, finding herself at age 62 eagerly anticipating a sumptuous future.

No one, not even her mother had made any attempt to prepare Sonia for what this stage of life would be like, but the indirect messages from all sides were loud and clear—once you're past those childbearing years, your sexual life is one long downhill slide. So she'd tried not to think too much about getting older. True, she had gone through some dramatic changes in the last ten years, and her life was definitely different from what it had been when she was caught up in mothering and working. Those had been good, fulfilling years, but this—this was a whole new world!

Menopause had not been an easy transition for Sonia—the night sweats, the grumpiness, the yeast infections, the memory loss, not to mention the vaginal dryness and loss of sexual desire. That whole fog had lifted a few years ago, and she had emerged in a much-altered body. She'd watched in astonishment as her smallish breasts had grown three sizes larger. She hadn't even known that bra sizes went beyond DD! The rest of her body had morphed into something she was only just now coming to recognize as her own. Monstrous curves had replaced her boyish hips. Even thinking about having intercourse with her former husband Ed had required buying bottles of gel designed to enhance her personal lubrication. And who needed one of those bikini waxes now that her butt had sagged and half of her graying pubic hair had fallen out, leaving her looking a bit like a plucked chicken?

And it wasn't simply the physical symptoms of the change of life that she'd endured. Relationships had ended and shifted. Her mother and dad, vigorously independent for many years, were suddenly no longer able to handle the upkeep of their home and had reluctantly accepted Sonia's help to move into an assisted-living facility. Then, Donna, Sonia's closest friend, was diagnosed with advanced ovarian cancer. The last year of Donna's life had been a nightmare that had left Sonia shaken and lonely.

All of this had happened against the background of her failed marriage to Ed, her partner of twenty-five years. Initially Ed was patient and affectionate even though Sonia's once-feverish passion had faded. But Viagra-equipped, he'd begun looking elsewhere, and their sex life had melted away, leaving them more companions than lovers. One unforgettable blustery day, Ed told her he'd fallen in love with a 38-year-old dance instructor who had the body and the sexual appetite he craved; the divorce had not been pretty.

It had been a long and uneven road that she'd traveled. She'd had to figure out who this newly single person was who had come to inhabit her graying body. Sonia's foray into therapy proved a valuable education; she'd learned a lot about herself and felt rewarded when she met a new, "emotionally available" guy at a Jewish Community

Center event. They were still trying to figure out what to call each other—"girlfriend and boyfriend" did not become them; "significant other" sounded manufactured. She was relishing a newfound intimacy that she hadn't known was possible in a relationship.

Sonia's sexual self-esteem had taken a battering from all the negative, degrading images of women her age that society had relegated to the sexual discard pile. But she had always been a fighter, and her instinct had been to reject the stereotypes and find her own way to grow older. With the proceeds of the divorce settlement and her Social Security payments in hand, she'd recently retired from her job as an administrative assistant. She didn't have it all figured out yet. But she was learning what gave her pleasure, what gave her pain, what helped her relax, and what helped restore her. Finally able to focus on her pottery, Sonia was seized with an energy and passion that made her laugh at the idea of being seen as over the hill and irrelevant. Who cared about smooth skin and a boyish figure when she had this hard-earned freedom?

By listening to and learning from the hundreds of dynamic and generous women like Sonia who contributed their remarkable stories to our work, we have reached the unambiguous conclusion that the loss of sexual vibrancy and self-esteem is *not* an inevitable consequence of growing old. Yes, sexy is different after 50. Desire waxes and wanes, illnesses and injuries impede our ability to engage in sexual activity, partners die or divorce us, and we wonder if it is truly possible to have low libido and still exude sexual self-confidence. But reconnecting with our sexual selves can lead us to an appreciation for the future. The pleasures we can anticipate enjoying into our 90s are not privileges granted only to the young but are rights that we older women need to seize with confidence. It's neither sinful nor sordid to have high desire, nor is it a crime to place the sex act itself in the past if that is what we choose.

This stage of life is full of potential, as Cindy, a 57-year-old from Dallas, says, "I think women over age 55 are experiencing the

> It's not just the physical stuff that gets in our way, but how we judge each other. Like there is one right way to grow old.
>
> —*Eileen, 58, Baltimore, Maryland*

natural effects of aging without being locked into them. We're all testing assumptions and limits... even though there are some limits that are natural and biological; it's the sociological and psychological ones that we can change."

Mature women have come to realize that youthful standards of sexiness no longer make sense, but a different body size and shape need not spell the end of intimacy. Bessie, a 60-year-old singer from Detroit, says, "I am expecting to continue to enjoy my sexuality, whatever my body is. I am not really ready to let it go. Although there is all this Viagra stuff, I don't want somebody who wants to have intercourse with me two or three times a day or ten times a week. I'd say, 'Go away!' I don't need that, I mean it is not part of who I am...when I was younger that was cool, not now—that just is not my thing. But I very much like it that every day my husband cherishes me, kisses me, hugs me, maybe even gets turned on by me. We are compatible sexually—two or three times a month we have intercourse or maybe some hands-on genital play. But every day we are touching and kissing each other. I am very blessed...I like to hold hands and he likes to hold hands. We truly want to lean into each other much more."

Bessie is one of a number of women we talked with who have a strong sense of sexual self-worth. They have learned to pay attention to themselves and respect their own needs. She told us, "Any feelings of desire depend so much on the balance you have in your life at any given day. I feel that you have to be very aware of your own body to have strong desires, also you have to be able to 'be in the present moment' and allow yourself the luxury of listening to your wants and feelings and those of your partner."

As Bessie implies, this phase of life requires drafting a new model of sexuality, one that more than likely includes adjustments and modifications. More than half of the women who responded to our survey said that indeed there had been a change in the level of their desire. But we also discovered that older women—even those in their 90s—continue to be interested in matters of the heart, and they report that their satisfaction with sex has not changed. As a matter of fact, the majority of women in our study who had a partner said they would like to have sex with that person significantly more often than they currently do.

Yet there are also periods in the life of nearly all older women when their desire for sex drops to the low end of the range, times when their energy is focused elsewhere. For example, Loretta, a long-time stay-at-home mom and grandmother, says, "I used to yearn for ultimate sexual fusion with my partner, but now the desire for that has faded away. My satisfaction comes from my spiritual life."

To be a mature woman in today's world is a very different prospect than it was for earlier generations. We can reasonably expect many more years of health and independence than could our mothers or certainly our grandmothers. And for those of us in the baby boom generation, the history of nearly unlimited options for occupation and educational direction has encouraged us to view the future as something we can mold according to our own preferences. Yet our sexual futures are rarely given serious consideration and even less often openly discussed. Unaccustomed to the loss of control over this part of our lives, we've begun a quest for some answers. Many women told us that they don't have it all together; they recognize that the next decades are uncharted territory, and few of them have any clear idea what to expect. Still, they do have hopes and dreams for their sexual futures, and we wanted to get a picture of what those look like. So we asked them.

Hopes and Dreams for Your
Sexual Future

Women have come to understand that the past is not necessarily a good predictor of the future, that circumstances and relationships are constantly in a state of flux. They're often a bit flabbergasted by the twists and turns their sexual lives have taken. For example, Alma, a divorced 55-year-old from the lower midwest who now shares her home and heart with another woman, told us, "Well I hope to stay with my partner. We were together five years, and then we were apart thirteen years, and now we are together again so we will celebrate our sixth anniversary soon. I want to continue to feel passion and desire and actually feel it as much or more than I did before. And I hope we continue to have sex even through the time that we are really old ladies. I am not sure how to put this but because of the experiences that I have had over the last years—a long period really of celibacy, even though I was in a partnership and not feeling interested in sex, and then rediscovering my sexual self—I am just really quite amazed at the waxing and waning of sexual desire."

In general, women over 50 expect a slight decrease in sexual desire over the next 10 years; at the same time, regardless of whether they are currently partnered or not, they expect that sex itself will be slightly more enjoyable for them. Eliza, a 55-year-old Christian educator from Alabama, offered the following comment: "Well, my hope is that I will have sexual desire until I die and that I will also have an intimate relationship with somebody up until I die. I don't see why I can't have both. Obviously if I get incapacitated I might not be able to have sex, but if I stay in good health and I am an active person and all of that I don't see why that wouldn't happen."

Across the country in eastern Oregon, Marlys, a 69-year-old who reconnected with the love of her life after her first husband died, is proof that Eliza's dream can become a reality. Marlys offered the following comment, "I think I am incredibly fortunate to find someone who cares about me and who I care about. We share common interests, and as an added bonus we enjoy each other sexually even after fifteen years. And we trust each other enough that we don't have to live together!"

But dozens of women in our study do look toward the future with confusion and some regret. They acknowledge that their sexual aging has been more difficult than they imagined. Somberly, Roxanne told us, "Although I'm 65, in my mind I am 35 years old and I am attracted to 35-year-olds. It is hard to be sexually attracted to people my age or older. I now understand how 'dirty old men' feel." Roxanne finds herself perplexed by these feelings, as she's always considered herself to be "age and sex appropriate" when it came to desire. Now she's facing an internal crisis, struggling to understand how to reconcile her feelings with her intention.

> The reality is for a majority of people that the spirit doesn't necessarily grow old, but the vehicles that we carry those spirits in age. For many that's a difficult situation. Your sexual desire may be there but your body can't quite get you there.
>
> —*Ginny, 63, Salt Lake City, Utah*

Roxanne's confusion is mirrored in the responses we received from widowed and divorced women whose visions for their sexual futures had always been populated by a loving partner. Older women who find themselves without a partner are often left straining to accept a different version of aging than the one they had been anticipating.

Many widowed and divorced women would like to have a long-term relationship but recognize it might not happen. Yet they are sexual beings whether in an intimate relationship or not. Cathy, a grandmother of seven, told us, "When I think about being in a relationship with someone—a life partner—there are many different kinds of relationships. There's companionship, sexual relationship, and I'm sure there are many other ways of people being together. For me, right now in my life, I'm torn between that companionship piece and the sexual piece. Can I find a relationship where I can have both?"

Emma's experiences with sexual desire have taught her that there are many benefits of patience and faith. She views the future optimistically, but always with a practical eye. Emma has been married three times. "I've been more unmarried than I have been married. And facing life singly with very few friends—maybe three girlfriends over the years—not having companionship is a sorrow or has been for me. But I'm evolving. Now I am bold enough not to give up and to become the character I want to be, trusting that I'll find my companion, and my sex mate."

After years of wandering through a wilderness of destructive relationships, Emma found herself alone again at 63. Her third husband died, and she decided to direct the changes in her life. "I wanted to do all the things I had not experienced as a teen. I'm living on SSI and my savings—not much—but I've taken every poetry class I can." Now 73 and "full of vinegar," she recently wrote to us that she has a new man in her life. She's eager to share her new passions and her life-long sensuality, but her hard-won self-esteem will not allow her to abandon her own goals for the sake of another relationship. As she's told us, "I'm enjoying being courted, but I'm not losing my head, or my financial independence!"

But any intimate relationship requires some compromises and adjustments, even those that have endured over many years. At this point in life, striking a new bargain with a long-time partner can seem like more work than it's worth, so many women have decided to just stay the course, at least for the foreseeable future.

Raylene, a 54 year-old attorney from Nevada, is trying to come to terms with how she and her husband will fare over the long term.

"Growing up Catholic, you learn early that you stay together whether you're compatible or not. Sure, I would like it if my husband and I were a little bit more in sync sexually, and other ways, too. We've talked about it some. And I don't see that happening in the near future unless I give up one of my many outside activities. I'd really rather not have

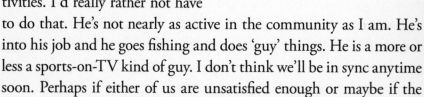

I prefer men to masturbation. I hope I never have to be without a partner. I know I can live without one but I hope that I never have to.

—*Karin, 62, Chattanooga, Tennessee*

to do that. He's not nearly as active in the community as I am. He's into his job and he goes fishing and does 'guy' things. He is a more or less a sports-on-TV kind of guy. I don't think we'll be in sync anytime soon. Perhaps if either of us are unsatisfied enough or maybe if the pressure is on some things might change, but I kind of doubt it."

Considering their hopes and dreams for the future leads many women beyond 50 to think about their own mortality and about their partners' life expectancy. Wendy, a golf pro from Arizona, told us, "You know, I was thinking that as we get into our 50s, we truly know we are getting older. You begin to wonder how long you're going to be around. I think my husband and I are going to be together for quite a while, but you never know. And I often think if something were to happen to my husband and I were left alone, a widow, I think I probably wouldn't remarry again. I don't see myself with anybody else. And yet I wouldn't want him to be alone. I mean I wouldn't want him to be alone really. It would be really hard for him."

Joyce, 58, who has been married for 39 years, knows about the realities of life and death and sustaining relationships first hand. Born in Milan, Italy, she and her family moved to the United States when she was a young girl. Joyce wants to emulate a friend who has stayed very strongly connected to her sensuality as she has aged. "I'd

> As time goes on, I don't have any specific hope and dreams for finding my soul mate. I've got my vibrator.
>
> —*Mabel, 65, Episcopalian, Burlington, Vermont*

like to age sexually like a friend of mine, may she rest in peace; I wish to God she were still alive. When we used to go anywhere, we'd follow the Italian custom— the men would sit in the front seat of the car and the women in the backseat. So there were three men in front and three girls in the back. And one time my friend, Colletta, who was 85 at the time, put her hands around her husband's shoulders and said, 'My husband, my lover, and my friend.' And I said, 'I have to ask you a question—you are probably going to think I am terrible—but do you still have sex with your husband?' She said, 'Until the day I die!' And that is my hope. I mean she was wonderful; they had such a great relationship. When my husband and I have any problems, I always remember that quote; 'my husband, my lover, and my friend' and she was married at the age of 14! It's amazing, they were married over sixty years when she passed away. To be like Colletta, that is my deepest wish."

Defining a New Sexual Reality

Joyce was fortunate to have found a role model whom she can use as a guide for her own sexual aging. Joyce recognizes that she, like the rest of us, is moving into an unpredictable time. There is simply no way to click on Mapquest and get a set of directions that will guide you to the smoothest, easiest, or happiest way for you to age sexually. The options are limitless, yet we are often unaware of the choices we have. The negative aspects of aging are generally much clearer to us than the positive ones. We know what we don't want, but we are frequently at a loss when it comes to labeling what we do want.

"I know I don't want to grow old like my mother—bitter and lonely," says Martha, "but I don't know how many women really embrace old age in a positive way. I want to be a happy old lady, but I'm not sure what that would mean for me." In some ways, we are all dreamers like Martha, tentatively approaching our sexual aging with vague hopes and more than a hint of skepticism. But rather than wander aimlessly toward old age, we can set a course that will allow us keep our sexual self-esteem healthy and vital.

1. **Examine your expectations and your world view.** Take a few minutes to go back to Chapter 1 and review the questions posed there. Consider the answers you gave before you had read this book. Would you give different responses now? Here are a couple of additional questions for you to address in light of what you have learned:

- What, if anything, do you want to do about boosting your sexual self-esteem?

- What choices are you making now that are helping you embrace the future?

2. **Cast off the images of older women's sexuality spun by the media and popular culture, and shift preconceived notions.** Together we can change the world and banish the stereotypes of older women's sexuality. Testing the limits and breaking through the barriers are often thought to be the province of the young. But those of us with experience and maturity have some tricks up our sleeves that can help us to do the same, and maybe do it with less angst. Fifty-five-year-old Esther told us, "I would like to nurture my sexuality. I definitely want to enjoy it. To savor it. Not a lot, just a little. No, I would like to savor it a lot. And I guess continue to

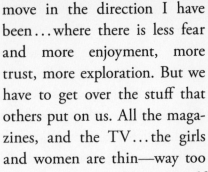

We don't see things as they are;
we see them as we are.
        —*Anaïs Nin*

move in the direction I have been...where there is less fear and more enjoyment, more trust, more exploration. But we have to get over the stuff that others put on us. All the magazines, and the TV...the girls and women are thin—way too thin and unrealistic—and it's all geared toward making yourself attractive to someone else. It's neither realistic nor attainable. I think that because we haven't had conversations about this more, expectations get in the way of real experiences."

3. **Learn about the range of normal experience and the choices you have for your sexual expression.** Understanding that sexual desire is unpredictable, especially once you are beyond 50, is an important step down the road to finding the version of mature sexuality that works for you. There is no "right way" to redefine your sexual self—it's an individual journey. Some women in our study were surprised to find a resurgence of their passion after years of marginally satisfying, routine sex. Others sought to reclaim their lost desire by seeking help from a therapist. Still others found that a prescription for bio-identical hormones or a testosterone patch was the answer for them. And some are analyzing the choices they've made to date and remaining open to possibilities.

Directing your attention toward valuing your uniqueness and away from judging yourself against some artificial standard will take you a long way down this path. You may never delight in your flabby upper arms, but you can certainly learn to ignore them in favor of savoring your rich capacity for warm, human connections.

Annette describes how her perspective has changed: "Well, I am in transition. I'm turning 60 and my whole body is changing. I'm beginning to see myself as an older person. My sexual desire is waning, and it's letting me know that I am aging appropriately. It is part of that whole ball of wax that goes along with my aching joints and my dimming eyesight, and even losing a few teeth. I'm seeking to accept this with grace."

Marnie is a successful businesswoman who has never married. She is content with her single life, but she isn't closing the door to other options. Now 61, she says, "I would want to continue to have a succession of intimate relationships, although if the right man came along at this point, I could imagine becoming committed to one person. I feel more settled down and less needy of having a variety of sexual experiences than I did before. I am a serial monogamist, not a woman who sleeps around. I really love my life so much, so I don't actively wish it was different." Marnie somewhat sheepishly confessed that she has been consciously wishing for a long-term intimate relationship for a while. "It is really a wish and not a preference. It is in no way an obsession. I would never compromise my values or standards to have it. And I have seen other women my age do that. Especially those who have really postponed marriage."

Unlike Marnie, most women in the United States have been married at some point. They have learned their desire is not static: it subsides and may swell again. Selma, 53, an avid horsewoman, sees rekindling the desire that is currently eluding her as a worthy goal and one within her reach. She told us, "Well, I don't know where it [desire] has gone... it has definitely gone somewhere. And I wonder if it just goes away or if you just don't have it very much anymore after menopause. I really wonder about that. My desire certainly seems to have been redirected—keeping things in order is such a priority for me now. After the terror of September 11, people had this great need for order; their lives were in chaos. And I felt that way too. I have always had a great need for order but I think it has been intensified since then. I'm trying to rethink this though. You know, relationships are really all I am going to take with me. And so that is what I really need to be working on. And certainly my sexual relationship with my husband is part of it. And so I think it is a matter of really redirecting. I need to pull it back out of cleaning the house or the design work that I am doing—or whatever else I am doing to fulfill my passion for prettiness and interior decorating. The wonderful look and feel I've created in my home, and the time I've expended to do that, I need to redirect that into my relationship. I can carry that with me. It will sustain me."

Alyce is another woman who understands sustaining relationships. Her sexual desire is high, but she hasn't had sex in a very long time. She is 62 and discovered about five years ago that her husband had been having affairs throughout their marriage. For economic and family reasons, she decided to stay married, at least for the foreseeable future. But the longing for something different is readily apparent. "Well I would love, I really would love to go into my older years with a different partner. Just holding hands and going for a walk or taking someone's arm and just being with them. I don't even have that. I sometimes think maybe he will die before I do and I will meet someone…this is a possibility you know. It may be we will agree at some point to separate and that is not out of the question because there are lots of days that I think we both wonder why we are together. People might judge my decision, but I've become very aware and very respectful of issues in people's lives that cause them to do what they do—and that affects the sex thing as well. If we were given the ideal life and everything went wonderfully well and all our needs are met, oh boy! We might be in great shape but there are very few people with that kind of life. I mean we are all very different as a result of all these different things. I just know deep in my heart that I would really love to have a loving sexual relationship. I get a great deal of comfort from my faith."

> I hope to find a long-term partner who is loving and sexual—someone to grow old with me. I have another half century to do that.
>
> —*Jenna, 54-year-old Midwesterner*

We heard a lot about how women had broadened the focus of their sexuality to include their connection to something sacred. Some find their spiritual needs can be met through self-improvement courses or through nondenominational retreats. Others recognize that their own faith interacts powerfully with their sexuality. As Jewel, a 52-year-old from Kansas City, told us, "I was reflecting as we were having this interview. It never dawned on me, when I knew I was going to be talking to you, how much my faith and my spiritual belief would come into this whole conversation. It really has had a profound affect."

4. **Become your own role model for sexual aging.** We may not set out to do it in a conscious way, but as women we have a tendency to seek out role models to act a guides, mentors, and even coaches as we face new challenges in life. If we are lucky, we know real people—women such as Colletta or maybe even our mothers or older sisters—who are willing to be candid with us about how they have handled their sexuality. More often than not, though, our role models are people we don't really know.

Leila's Manifesto for Sexual Self-Esteem

I am…

• More than the sum of all of my accomplishments.

• More than any measure of my appearance.

• The container of my own ideal—she's inside me.

• The definer of my own allure.

• My own soulmate—and a first-rate friend and companion.

• Comfortable with my sexual wisdom.

• Able to redirect my sexual energy wherever I want.

• Able to define the kind of intimacy I want.

• Able to leave a positive sexual legacy for future generations.

—Leila, 56, Cleveland, Ohio

Rather, they are women we see through the lens of the media and who possess certain appealing characteristics that resonate for us.

We asked women to name female celebrities, writers, poets, or teachers who were their role models for sexual aging. We collected a long list of names from Imogene Cunningham ("Her loving, but totally erotic photos capture the essence of desire and passion") to Cher ("Cher pops into my mind first. I hesitate to say that, because she's pretty controversial, and has had so much plastic surgery. But she really seems to be a woman who is really tuned into her sexuality. I have to admire her honestly for who she is"). The list included a host of others, from Angela Lansbury to Maya Angelou. As Annie told us, "Maya Angelou would definitely be on my list of role models. She is a very insightful woman and has had a lot of experiences. I don't know if forward and progressive are the right terms but she has always been pretty frank about her life, including her sexual life. She is pretty nonjudgmental about people."

Women saw admirable characteristics in these celebrities even though their knowledge of these women was generally based on the characters they portrayed on TV or in the movies or *People* magazine's take on their life. It is the qualities that they admire, whether actually possessed by the women they named or not, that reflect what women want for themselves. Consider how Marcie described Susan Sarandon—one of the most often mentioned role models for sexual aging: "She is someone I admire greatly. I love her to death. She is honest and intelligent. She is beautiful but not trying to look thirty years younger than she is. She is talented and she is very much involved in all kinds of causes. She is just a fabulous woman. She is great role model for me."

In general, positive role models are conduits for helping us recognize what we appreciate in ourselves. When we identify with celebrities we tend to do what Marcie has done with Susan Sarandon: we use the bits we know about them and create an image that fits our ideals. It is, in fact, our own values that we see mirrored in the women we most admire. Our role models may be celebrities whose lives do not look anything like our own, but the personal qualities that make them attractive to us really say more about us than about them.

There may not be any one individual who possesses all the qualities you seek in a role model for sexual aging, but each woman you admire for her strength of character, her comfort with her body, her emotional clarity, or her spiritual connectedness can shine a light on a part of you that deserves your attention and respect. Sexual self-esteem is a result of accumulating the wisdom to appreciate your own womanhood in its many aspects.

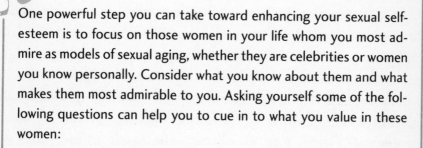

One powerful step you can take toward enhancing your sexual self-esteem is to focus on those women in your life whom you most admire as models of sexual aging, whether they are celebrities or women you know personally. Consider what you know about them and what makes them most admirable to you. Asking yourself some of the following questions can help you to cue in to what you value in these women:

1. What is her attitude toward sexuality and aging? How would she express that?

2. Is sex an important aspect of her life now? In the past?

3. How does she cope with changes in her level of sexual desire?

4. How does she cope with changes in her body's appearance?

5. How important are her intimate, e.g., sexual or potentially sexual, relationships?

6. How important are her relationships with other women in her life?

Remembering that the characteristics we most admire in others are reflections of ourselves, consider those attributes of positive sexual aging that you share with your role model. You can make this experience even more meaningful for yourself by actually writing out a list of these qualities. It may be a short list at first—that self-critical voice can be stubborn initially—but by naming our strengths out loud, we bolster our self-esteem. "I think of myself as pretty gutsy these days," says Barbara, "There's not much that hurts my feelings. I've always admired those women who can stand up and ask for what they want without worrying about how others are going to react to them. Well, I can do that now. There is definitely a connection between being assertive and feeling good about yourself sexually. I didn't get that when I was younger."

5. **Be intentional.** Once you have created your own role model for sexual aging, take some time to consider how you can translate this model into a real, living, breathing example. Step away from your normal routine, and take some time out to truly focus. To do so, use any of a number of techniques wise women use to calm and relax their minds. For some, it's getting a massage or learning silent meditation. Others turn to a more active form, utilizing yoga or Pilates or dance. Some use prayer. Jewish women may invoke the concept of *kavanah,* a Hebrew word that is often translated as "concentration," "devotion," or "intent," as a useful technique. Kavanah, which is actually a mind-set for prayer, is a way of focusing that helps turn rote words into meaningful worship. Regardless of the particular method you use to get there, the goal is to become deliberate and contemplative. This process can help you overcome mundane distractions and aid you in recognizing how those worn-out old tapes—the negative self-talk and the limiting images of older women—cloud your view. By shutting them out, you can begin to clarify your vision of a sexual future that makes sense for you.

Cindy is a 52-year-old Native American who finds that her tradition has helped her blossom into a wise elder. "The women in my culture are great teachers. From them I've learned to respect myself." Cindy continued, "My sexual desire is probably not going to get much higher in the future but it is probably not going to be totally diminished either. The desire really is up to the individual. I think my desire could be higher. I think I could certainly do things. I could read erotic books; I could dance; I could watch movies; I could, you know masturbate. I could do many things to heighten my desire—but my life seems to be full without having to come to that peak, that high sexual peak. I just choose not to.

"I used to think that keeping a husband meant I had to be a beautiful, sexually alluring, Victoria's Secret kind of person. But I just don't feel that my sexual self is dependent on having a man constantly desiring me. I don't have to dress up in just the right little black dress and play provocative games. I can if I want to, but I call the shots now. I am conscious that I am becoming a more focused and spiritual person. I'm looking forward to a time when I can express these thoughts to more than just a few people. They might be surprised what is lurking under my sweatband."

6. **Refocus on self-acceptance.** Natalie, the woman in Chapter 3 whose husband hid his homosexuality from her and their children for years, is coming to terms with her decisions. "I guess as a young woman I wished I had known much more about myself before getting married. I wish that I would have had more of a close intimate, passionate, caring life with a partner. I'm learning to accept my role in this drama, and am wondering where the next phase of my life will lead."

Cecelia, a talkative, upbeat woman of 66 who participated in one of our workshops, is also wondering what is next for her. She doesn't want her past to get in the way. Cecelia described her life as one of struggle with intimate relationships. A single mother, she related how frustrating it was to find a partner during the time her kids were growing up. "I had way too much baggage and ended up being pretty needy. Men simply ran the other way. For a long time I couldn't see that I was partly responsible. Conquering some of my demons—like coming to terms with my weight and with the size of my paycheck—is real important to me." Now, she's begun to see the world as a place of fullness and possibilities. As part of an exercise for identifying a sexual future for herself, she wrote:

I am not just the sum of—

• My age.

• My cup, weight, or dress size— nor my appearance, wrinkles, or back fat.

• My checkbook balance.

• My driving record.

• My memory.

• My hot flashes and sleep disturbances—or the number of hours I sleep a night.

• My blood pressure and heart rate.

• The number of aches and pains I have.

• How successful my children are.

• The number of grandkids I have.

• My level of sexual desire/sex drive/appetite.

• The number of sexual partners I have had.

As Cecelia's affirmations demonstrate, an older woman can create a whole new sexual profile for herself. And we know lots of them who are doing just that. They're discarding the old patterns that have left them wanting and are weaving a new tapestry. Whether by prolonged introspection or sudden catharsis, they are redesigning their own vision of their sexual future. In doing so, they are dissolving the shroud of silence that has so long surrounded the subject of sexuality in older women and freeing following generations from the limitations of conventional images of aging and sexuality.

Creating a Legacy

Many women spoke to us about wanting to leave a legacy for younger women and men in their lives that will encourage them to envision the sexuality of their older years with optimism. They want to pass down their own stories, their hopes, love, wishes, advice, and blessings for healthy sexual aging. There is a way to break the chain of negativity and myth and to give our children and grandchildren the healthy and realistic roadmap that has been missing for older women for so long.

As Ursula, who lives on an island off the Maine Coast, says, "What I want is to continue going! There are some days that go by when I think, 'Oh, Lord, if I can just get through this day I will be very happy.' I want to be able to keep writing, keep feeling positive about my life, be there for my lover, for my grandchildren now, and later. My mother and my grandmother were not able to be there for me, but just maybe I can be there for the next generation and the next after that."

If you'd like to bequeath a legacy of positive sexual aging to your heirs, there is no time like the present to begin. It all starts with you—and how much you want to leave. Margaret encouraged us to tell women, even if it might sound like a cliché, that "We are a powerful force. When our health is optimum, our sexual energy directed and available, our gifts and talents give passion and meaning to our lives. Not only are we available to do what we are called to do in this lifetime, we'll be leaving these gifts to the next generation. From what I can tell (and I turn 60 this year) the best is yet to come!"

Mature women have the charisma, courage, and capacity to alter the culture not only for themselves but over the course of the next century. Is it hard to imagine a future where women's sexual self-esteem is bathed in the light of authenticity, autonomy, and assertiveness? As you move into the rest of your life, we invite you to consider three things you can do to assure that our great-great-granddaughters can take their sexual self-esteem for granted.

1. Create an environment for speaking the unspoken truths.

As we become clearer about who we are, and as we become role models for others, we are more prepared to bequeath our legacy. If we had all been blessed with sexually confident, honest, communicative older women who had guided us through our development, the task of passing on the guidance we received to the next generation would, perhaps, come more easily to us. Few of us have been so lucky, but that does not mean we don't have much of value to give to our sons and daughters.

One aspect of sexual health and well-being for women beyond 50 is the recognition of our capacity to powerfully influence others. We all know how to make small talk and can chat endlessly about the little things in life. Now, it is time to speak out about one of life's big things: sex and aging. You'll increase the odds that you will improve your own sexual self-esteem by doing so, and you'll begin to convey your unique experience to others.

The experience Gloria shared with us brought this point home very poignantly. Her 83-year-old mother, Hilda, was surprised to be asked to participate in a study about sexual desire. Reading the survey caused her to realize that she had not acknowledged her own needs for much of her married life. When Hilda was young, her mother had discouraged her from attending to her own desires. Now Hilda realized that she had probably passed on the same negative message to her offspring. She called her 45-year-old daughter Gloria and invited her to coffee. The two women had the first open conversation about adult sexuality they had ever had. Gloria was deeply grateful for her mother's candor, and they began a dialogue about ending the pattern of generations of women in their family who had not acknowledged their own sexual desires. Hilda now has hopes that her granddaughters will be positively impacted.

You can tap into the generative power of others by providing opportunities for women to gather simply to talk about sexual aging. We discovered that our "What color is your sexual desire?" house gatherings offered women one of the first chances they'd ever had to talk about their own sexuality in a relaxed, informal group setting. If you're able to keep the culture of the group nonjudgmental, you'll hear all kinds of stories. The paths women travel are amazingly diverse. We've discovered that once you open the door, those who enter the first time will clamor for more. Don't be surprised if the group wants to continue talking on a regular basis. As one of the hostesses wrote to us several weeks after we met with a group of her fabulous friends, "Since you guys can't come back every week, we're going to try to do it on our own. We want to keep talking about our sex lives. That one night wasn't enough—you just got us started."

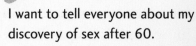

I want to tell everyone about my discovery of sex after 60.

—*Sadie, Jewish divorcee, New Jersey*

You might consider expanding on this concept by creating a forum or salon or women's circle where older and younger women mix and mingle for the expressed purpose of passing on sexual wisdom. Think about hosting a mother/daughter potluck that gives women a chance to tell their stories in a safe, comfortable environment where everyone can be themselves. In such a setting, each woman can begin to be a catalyst to help other women chart their own course.

2. Encourage others to choose their own direction for sexual aging.

Connie, a 71-year-old account executive, has been considering how her actions will impact her offspring. "As a younger person my own sexuality was a bit of a mystery to me. Learning how to express that side of me—both to myself and to a partner—was more complicated than I had imagined. I had so much to learn...and of course there were certain performance skills that had to go with it. But now I know that other skills, human skills, communication skills are vital. There was this body of knowledge about human sexuality that I had to learn because it was not transmitted directly by my parents or by the school system. As I have aged, and developed additional wisdom and knowledge, my expressions of sexuality—or is it sensuality?— have shifted. Now, it's not that hard to talk to my husband about what sex means to him, how much he wants, how much I want, how much is enough, or if we even want to have any sex at this stage in our lives. But the real test for me is that I've begun talking to my friends about it much more often, and I don't think my grandkids will be immune to my musings either. I wish I could be around to see how they'll handle their sexuality when they are my age."

Your sexual choices can have resonance for the next generation and those who follow. As part of the potent and vital sisterhood of older women, your influence on the attitudes of younger women and of your peers is significant. By exuberantly modeling sexual self-esteem, you become an inspiration and light the way for others.

3. Celebrate!

Ceremony and ritual in our culture have usually been reserved to mark significant moments in our lives—the birth of a child, graduation, marriage, and death. Creating a new observance—one that celebrates mature sexual aging—can help us transform our culture, even if it's only one person at a time. We'd like to introduce you to Sophie, a courageous pianist of 59, who had been a popular, beloved day-care supervisor. She told us how, at the age of 50, when her youngest daughter left for college, she decided to resign from her position to find a new mission. What she discovered was something that many older women can relate to. Calling upon her friends and relatives for strength, she engaged upon a journey that took her to many corners of the United States. She hooked up with long-lost neighbors and laughed long into the night with her old college roommates. They fortified her as she contemplated her next move. But then, she decided to do something that few women have ever done. "One postmenopausal day, after many years of floundering to understand my beyond 50 self, I finally realized that I had 'reentered' the world on my own terms—with clearer boundaries, better health, keener perceptions." Sophie, with great intent, decided to mark the moment by hosting a gathering with a group of her closest women friends and her two adult daughters, "those who have supported me on my journey thus far."

Responding to a glittering invitation, 20 women, some festooned in silk and satin and others in cotton and spangled flip-flops, joined together in Sophie's living room. High on a cliff overlooking the Pacific Ocean, they came to celebrate Sophie's emergence from her menopausal cocoon to hear her declare that she was a "sparkling, seasoned woman." Sophie explained to us that she'd taken an almost mythical inward journey and had unloaded her "accumulated baggage, returning to the 'outer world' lighter" and on her own terms. "I returned liberated, but there has been a fairly major shift in how I am in the world, and my major, intimate relationship has been profoundly affected. I know this shift is not a destination but part of an unfolding journey. I am redefining the role of the sexy older woman—and reclaiming the rest of my life. My somewhat astonished, caring daughters (one a physician and one a nurse) represent the future. The legacy I bequeath to them is that all women can be delightful, sexual beings." Using thread, beads, and feathers, the women present at her celebration each fashioned one piece of "fringe" that Sophie and her daughters have hung on a flowing, silken vest. Sophie told us, "I intend to wear it for years to come, and I'm going to leave it to my granddaughters so they'll know their grandmother as a woman of deep passion and deep convictions." Savoring the chocolate-covered strawberries and drinking champagne, the women toasted Sophie just as the sun set over the ocean. "I know that taking a moment to celebrate my sexual self doesn't mean that I am done unfolding from the cocoon, but that I am choosing a path of self discovery, sharing, growing, and searching for the peace that comes from a balance of giving and receiving." We salute Sophie for her remarkable creativity. And we encourage you to emulate her ritual— or better, yet design one of your own. Be it a quiet pat on your own back for having the courage to step out on a new path, or a big party honoring your shift in being in the world, celebrate yourself.

Bon Voyage

It is well past time to take a long look over the tops of our bifocals and focus on altering our culture. Through reflection, through opening connections, through learning more about the holistic nature of women's sexuality and self-confidence beyond 50, we know we can transform our society from an adherence to mythology about aging sexuality in the older women to a recognition of the full spectrum of possibility. Hollywood, the TV talk shows, and the popular press need to discard their tired old images and to see older women for who we are and what we are. It is time for women beyond 50 to seize control of the picture of aging female sexuality so predominant in our society. It is time we reframe our inner conversations and blaze the trail for younger generations of women and men. It is time to throw back the covers and expose to the world the power, vitality, and creativity of real women growing older with their sexual self-esteem intact, and prepared to do so on their own terms. Contrary to popular opinion, we're not over the hill, but rather comin' round the mountain. Transcending the sexual scripts we've written for ourselves and the ones others have written for us is an ongoing journey. As older women in today's society, we have options previous generations never envisioned, and we are facing challenges they never imagined. Talking to one another, to our partners, to our children, and to our health-care providers about our sexuality can aid us all. We can gain greater understanding of the sexual realities of the older woman—not only for ourselves but as a legacy for our daughters and nieces and granddaughters. Leaving a sexual legacy that pairs hope with affirmation is not only possible but imperative. Our hats go off to the women we've spoken to, the women who so generously gave us their time. May their thoughts, their actions, their laughter—and their legacy—become a rallying cry for us all. Perhaps Patty, a 55-year-old "student for life" said it best.

"An honest and forgiving nature, a beaming smile, a soul that seeks divinity. Compassion for children, a body fit enough to hike all day, a certain naughtiness. Clean teeth. Intimacy without the drama, without the raw vulnerability, like a slow dance to the Platters' 'Smoke Gets in Your Eyes'—exclusive, rhythmic, and more of a sweet surprise than a longing. I want my kids and their kids to know all of this. That's what matters now."

Bibliography

Books

Achterberg, Jeanne. *Women as Healer.* Boston: Shambala Publications, Inc., Random House, Inc., 1991.

Adams, Mike. *The Five Habits of Health Transformation.* E-book, online Truth Publishing.com, 2004.

Bakos, Susan Crain. *Still Sexy: How the Boomers Are Doing It.* New York: St. Martin's Press, 1999.

Baumeister, RF, and Tice DM. *The Social Dimension of Sex.* Boston: Allyn and Bacon, 2001.

Berman, Jennifer, M.D., and Laura Berman, Ph.D. *For Women Only: A Revolutionary Guide to Reclaiming Your Sex Life.* New York: Henry Holt, First Owl, 2002.

Blank, Joani, ed. *Still Doing It: Women and Men over 60.* San Francisco: Down There Press, 2000.

Blank, Joani, and Ann Whidden. *Good Vibrations: The Complete Guide to Vibrators.* San Francisco: Down There Press, 2000.

Brick, Peggy, and Jan Lunquist. *New Expectations: Sexuality Education for Mid and Later Life.* New York: SIECUS (Sexuality Information and Education Council of the United States), 2003.

Butler, Robert, N., M.D., and Myrna I Lewis, Ph.D. *The New Love and Sex After 60,* New York: Random House, Ballantine, 2002.

Cone, Faye Kitchener. *Making Sense of Menopause: Over 150 Women and Experts Share Their Wisdom, Experience, and Commonsense advice.* New York: Simon & Schuster, Fireside, 1993.

De Angelis, Barbara. *What Women Want Men to Know.* New York: Hyperion, 2001.

De Beauvoir, Simone. *The Second Sex.* New York: Bantam Books by arrangement with Alfred A. Knopf, Inc., 1970.

Ferrare, Cristina. *Okay, So I Don't Have a Headache.* New York: St. Martin's, 2000.

Fine, Stuart W., M.D., F.A.C.S., and Brenda D. Adderly, M.H.A. *The Libido Breakthrough: A Doctor's Guide to Restoring Sexual Vigor and Peak Health.* Los Angeles: Newstar, 1999.

Foley, Sallie, M.S.W, Sally A. Kope, M.S.W., and Dennis P. Sugrue, Ph.D. *Sex Matters for Women: A Complete Guide to Taking Care of Your Sexual Self.* New York: The Guilford Press, 2002.

Friday, Nancy. *Women on Top.* New York: Simon & Schuster, Pocket Books, 1991.

Fuchs, Estelle, Ph.D. *The Second Season.* New York: Doubleday, Anchor Press, 1978.

Furman, Friday Kerner. *Facing the Mirror: Older Women and Beauty Shop Culture.* New York: Routledge, 1997.

Goldstein, Andrew, and Marianne Brandon. *Reclaiming Desire: 4 Keys to Finding Your Lost Libido.* New York: Rodale with St. Martin's Press, 2004.

Gordon, Sol, and Elaine Fantle Shimberg. *Another Chance for Love: Finding a Partner Later in Life.* Avon, MA: Adams Media, 2004.

Gottman, John M., Ph.D., and Nan Silver. *The Seven Principles for Making Marriage Work.* New York: Three Rivers Press, 1999.

Harris, Maria. *Jubilee Time: Celebrating Women, Spirit, and the Advent of Age.* New York: Bantam Books, Doubleday Dell Publishing Group, 1995.

Hite, Shere. *The Hite Report.* New York: Dell Publishing, 1976.

Jacobowitz, Ruth S. *150 Most-Asked Questions About Midlife Sex, Love & Intimacy: What Women and Their Partners Really Want to Know.* New York: William Morrow and Co., 1995.

Jean-Murat, Carolle. *Menopause Made Easy: How to Make the Right Decisions for the Rest of Your Life.* Carlsbad, CA: Hay House, 1999.

Jones, Michael. *Creating an Imaginative Life.* Boston: Conari Press, 1995.

Juska, Jane. *A Round-Hilled Woman: My Late-Life Adventures in Sex and Romance.* New York: Villard, 2003.

Kaschak, Ellyn, and Leonore Tiefer, eds. *A New View of Women's Sexual Problems.* Binghamton, New York: The Haworth Press, Inc., 2001.

Kilbourne, Jean. *Can't Buy My Love: How Advertising Changes the Way We Think and Feel.* New York: Touchstone, Simon & Shuster, 2000.

Landau, Carol, Ph.D., Michele G. Cyr, M.D., and Anne W. Moulton, M.D. *The New Truth About Menopause.* New York: Penguin Putnam, Perigee, 1994.

Laumann, E. O., Gagnon, J. H., Michael, R. T., & Michaels, S. *The Social Organization of Sexuality: Sexual Practices in the United States.* Chicago: University of Chicago Press, 1994.

Laux, Marcus, N.D., and Christine Conrad. *Natural Woman, Natural Menopause.* New York: HarperCollins, 1997.

Macdonald, Barbara, with Cynthia Rich. *Look Me in the Eye: Old Women, Aging, and Ageism.* Denver: Spinsters Ink Books, 2001.

Malucci, Terri, ed. *Menopause Pink: Mid-Life Reflections of Wisdom and Humor.* Boulder, CO: Creativa Press, 2000.

Masters, William H., M.D., and Virginia E. Johnson. *Human Sexual Response.* New York: Little, Brown and Company, 1966.

Mead, Margaret. *Sex and Temperament in Three Primitive Societies.* New York: New American Library, William Morrow & Company Inc., 1950.

Monique Truong. *The Book of Salt.* Boston: Houghton Mifflin, 2003.

Muscio, Inga. *Cunt: A Declaration of Independence.* Emeryville, CA: Seal Press, 2002.

Northrup, Christiane. M.D. *The Wisdom of Menopause.* New York: Bantam Books, 2003.

———*Women's Bodies, Women's Wisdom: Creating Physical and Emotional Health and Healing, Completely Revised and Updated.* New York: Bantam Books, 1998.

Ogden, Gina, Ph.D. *Women Who Love Sex: An Inquiry into the Expanding Spirit of Women's Erotic Experience.* Cambridge, MA: Womenspirit Press, 1999.

Ojeda, Linda, Ph.D. *Menopause Without Medicine: Feel Healthy, Look Younger, Live Longer.* Alameda, CA: Hunter House, 1992.

Parker, William, H., M.D., Amy E. Rosenman, M.D., and Rachel Parker. *The Incontinence Solution: Answers for Women of All Ages.* New York: Simon & Schuster, 2002.

Petersen, James R. *The Century of Sex.* New York: Grove Press, 1999.

Pogrebin, Letty Cottin. *Getting Over Getting Older: An Intimate Journey.* New York: Little, Brown and Company, 1996.

Price, Joan. *Better Than I Ever Expected: Straight Talk about Sex After Sixty.* Emeryville, CA: Seal Press, 2006.

Reichman, Judith, M.D. *I'm Not in the Mood*. New York: William Morrow, First Quill, 1998.

Reinisch, June M., Ph.D., with Ruth Beasley, M.L.S. *The Kinsey Institute New Report on Sex*. New York: St. Martin's Press, 1990.

Roundtree, Cathleen. *On Women Turning 50, Celebrating Mid-Life Discoveries*. New York: HarperCollins, 1993.

Sang, Barbara, Joyce Warshow, and Adrienne J. Smith, eds. *Lesbians at Midlife: The Creative Transition*. Gardena, CA: Spinsters, Inc., 1991.

Savage, Linda E. *Reclaiming Goddess Sexuality: The Power of the Feminine Way (rev)*. Encinitas, CA: Divine Feminine Publications, 2004.

Schiff, Isaac, M.D. *Menopause: The Most Comprehensive, Up-to-Date Information Available to Help You*. New York: Three Rivers Press, 1996.

Schnarch, David, Ph.D. *Resurrecting Sex*. New York: HarperCollins, Quill, 2003.

Seaman, Barbara, and Gideon Seaman, M.D. *Women and the Crisis in Sex Hormones*. New York: Bantam Books by arrangement with Rawson Associates Publishers, 1979.

Sheehy, Gail. *Menopause: The Silent Passage*. New York: Pocket Books, Simon & Schuster, Inc., 1998.

Sichel, Deborah, M.D., and Jeanne Watson Driscoll, M.S., R.N., C.S. *Women's Moods: What Every Woman Must Know About Hormones, the Brain, and Emotional Health*. New York: HarperCollins, First Quill, 2000.

Some, Sobonfu. *The Spirit of Intimacy*. New York: William and Morrow, First Quill, 2000.

Somers, Suzanne. *The Sexy Years*. New York: Crown Publishers, 2004.

Steinem, Gloria. *Revolution from Within*. New York: Little Brown and Company, 1993.

Swartz, Susan. *Juicy Tomatoes: Plain Truths, Dumb Lies and Sisterly Advice About Life After 50*. Oakland: New Harbinger, 2000.

Tiefer, Leonore. *Sex Is Not a Natural Act, Second Edition*. Boulder, CO: Westview Press, Perseus Books Group, 2004.

Vanzant, Iyanla. *In the Meantime: Finding Yourself and the Love You Want*. New York: Fireside, Simon & Schuster, 1999.

Weed, Susan S. *Menopausal Years the Wise Woman Way*. Woodstock, NY: Ash Tree Publishing, 1992.

Westheimer, Dr. Ruth. *Sex After 50: Revving up Your Romance, Passion, and Excitement*. Sanger, CA: Quill Driver Press, 2005.

Winks, Cathy, and Anne Semans. *The Good Vibrations Guide to Sex, Third Edition*. San Francisco: Cleis Press, Inc. 2002.

Journals and Periodicals

Anderson, Garnet L., et al of The Women's Health Initiative Steering Committee, "Effects of Conjugated Equine Estrogen in Postmenopausal Women With Hysterectomy: Randomized Controlled Trial," *JAMA*. 291 no. 14 (2004):1701–1712.

Barclay, Laurie M.D., "Voice Changes Common During Menopause," *Menopause*. 11 (2004):151–158.

Bancroft, J., J. Loftus, J. Scott Long, "Distress about sex: a national survey of women in heterosexual relationships," *Archives of Sexual Behavior*. 32 (2003): 193–208.

Basson, R, "The female sexual response: a different model," *Journal of Sexual and Marital Therapy*. 26 no. 1 (2000):51–65.

———, "Introduction to special issue on women's sexuality and outline of assessment of sexual problems," *Menopause*. 11 no. 6 (2004): 709–713.

———, "A Model of Women's Sexual Arousal," *Journal of Sexual and Marital Therapy*. 28 (2002) 1–10.

Basson, R, Berman, J, Burnett, A, et al. "Report of the international consensus development conference on female sexual dysfunction: definitions and classifications," *Journal of Urology*. 163 no. 3 (2000):888–93.

Bond, C.M., "Unleashing Your Libido: An Effort in Honesty, Time and Determination," *Seattle Woman*, February 2005, 11–15.

Buvat, J., "Androgen therapy with dehydroepiandrosterone," *World Journal of Urology*. 21 no. 5 (2003):346–55.

Cahill, Sean, Ken South, and Jane Spade, "Outing Age, Public Policy Issues Affecting Gay, Lesbian, Bisexual and Transgender Elders," Policy Institute of the National Gay and Lesbian Task Force Foundation, 2000.

Davis, Susan R., Sonia L. Davison, Susan Donath, and Robin J. Bell, "Circulating Androgen Levels and Self-reported Sexual Function in Women" *JAMA*. vol. 294, no. 1, July 6, 2005, 91–96.

Deer, Brian, "Love Sickness," *London Sunday Times Magazine*. 28, September 2003.

Dennerstein, L, Lehert, P, and Dudly, E, "Short Scale to Measure Female Sexuality: Adapted from McCoy Female Sexuality Questionnaire," *Journal of Sex and Marital Therapy*. 27 (2001):339–351.

Farrington, Arin, "Female Sexual Health in Midlife and Beyond: Addressing Female Sexual Distress," *Health and Sexuality, A Publication of the Association of Reproductive Health Professionals.* vol. 10, no. 2, July 2005, 3–16.

Ganz, P.A., et al. "Quality of Life in Long-Term, Disease-Free Survivors of Breast Cancer: A Follow-up Study," *Journal of the National Cancer Institute.* 94 no. 1 (2002): 39–49.

Ghosh, Pallab, "Low Self-Esteem 'Shrinks Brain'," *BBC News,* UK edition, 20 November, 2003.

Healy, Melissa, "Girlfriend Power," *The Seattle Times.* June 15, 2005, from *Los Angeles Times.*

Jiroutek, M.R., C.C., Johnston, and C. Longcope, "Changes in Reproductive Hormones and SHBG in a Group of Postmenopausal Women Measured Over 10 Years: Menopause." *Journal of the North American Menopause Society.* 5 (1998): 90–94.

Koch, Patricia Barthalow, and Phyllis Kernoff; "Facing the Unknown: Social Support During the Menopausal Transition," *Women and Therapy.* 3/3/2004, vol. 27, 3/4, ISSN: 0270-3149.

Laumann, E.O., A. Paik, and RC Rosen, "Sexual dysfunctions in the United States; prevalence and predictors" *JAMA.* 28 (1999): 537–544.

Merkin, Daphne, The Way We Live Now: 3-6-05; A Fairy Tale for grown-ups *The New York Times Magazine,* March 6, 2005.

Nappi, R. E., et al, "Climacteric Complaints, Female Identity, and Sexual Dysfunctions," *Journal of Sex and Marital Therapy.* 27 (2001): 567–576.

Nicolosi A, EO Laumann, DB Glasser, et al. "Sexual Behavior and Sexual Dysfunctions After Age 40: The Global Study of Sexual Attitudes and Behaviors," *Urology* 2004; 64: 991–997.

Sell, Randall L, "Defining and Measuring Sexual Orientation: A Review," *Archives of Sexual Behavior,* vol. 26, no. 6 (1997) : 643–658.

Shrifen, Jan L; Glenn D. Braunstein, James A. Simon, Peter R. Casson, John E. Bustert, Geoffrey P. Redmond, Regula E. Burki, Elizabeth S. Ginsburg, Raymond C. Rosen, Sandra R. Leiblum, Kim E. Caramelli, Norman A. Maser, Kirtley P. Jones, and Claire A. Daugherty, "Transdermal Testosterone Treatment in Women with Impaired Sexual Function After Oophorectomy." *The New England Journal of Medicine.* September 7, 2000 (10), 343: 682–688.

Tiefer, Leonore, "The Selling of 'Female Sexual Dysfunction'," *Journal of Sex and Marital Therapy.* 27 (2001): 625–628.

Tomlinson, John, "Taking a sexual history," *British Medical Journal.* 317 (1998): 1573–1576.

Online Articles

Conboy, Lisa, E. O'Connell, and A. Domar, "Quality of Life Study: Perimenopause/Menopause, Women at Mid-life: Symptoms, Attitudes, and Choices An Internet Based Survey," womens-health.com/research_center/qol_result.html.

Dennerstein, L., "Female Androgen Deficiency Syndrome: Definition, Diagnosis, and Classification: An International Consensus Conference," *MedscapePortals Inc.,* www.medscape.com.

Greenberg, Richard, *"The Olympics and Kavanah"* www.aish.com/spirituality/prayer, October 5, 2000.

Hamilton, Eleanor, "Body Image and Aging: Learning to Love the Changes in Love," www.grandtimes.com/bodyimage.html.

Hoffman, Heather, Ph.D., "Re-examining Sexual Desire," www.FemalePatient.com/sexualhealth.

Mazer, Norman A., M.D., Ph.D. "Effect of ERT on testosterone levels in women: Differences between oral and transdermal routes of administration," OBG Management Online, copyright 2005, Dowden Health Media, www.obgmanagement.com.

Newshe Patient Experience Survey. www.newshe.com/survey.shtml.

Smith, Heather, "Don't let arthritis spoil your sex life," National Association of Senior Friends, ehc.healthegate.com/GetContent.asp?siteid-1CA14AB-79CD-11D4-81F3-00508B1.

Tay Boon Lin, "Sexuality and the Menopause: Geneva Foundation for Medical Education and Research," First Consensus Meeting on Menopause in East Asian Region. www.gfmer.ch/Book/bookmp/48.htm.

Wilson, Richard C., "Can Your Heart Handle Sex?" National Association of Senior Friends, ehc.healthegate.com/GetContent.asp?siteid-1CA14AB-79CD-11D4-81F3-00508B1.

Women Health Interactive, "Midlife Sexuality, Make It an Adventure," *Midlife Health Center.,* womens-health.com/health_center/meidle/sex_advent.html.

Website Citations

www.101sexualhealth.com

www.aarp.org

www.apa.org

www.arhp.org (Association of Reproductive Health Professionals)

www.breastcancer.org

www.cancer.org

www.clitical.com

www.fsd-alert.org

http://factfinder.census.gov

www.human-dynamics.com

www.insiders.connection.com

www.lifeclinic.com/focus/diabetes/sex.as

www.LifeMD.com

www.MayoClinic.com

www.newshe.com

www.pdrhealth.com

www.seniorfriends.org

www.seniorhealth.about.com/od/safesex/a/AIDS_seniors.htm

www.seniorSex.org

www.sexsupport.org/aging.html

www.sexualhealth.com

www.StrokeAssociation.org

Helpguide, a project of the Rotary Club of Santa Monica and the Center for Healthy Aging: www.helpguide.org

Hysterectomy Linked to Elevated Heart Disease Risk: www.medscape.com/viewarticle/501739

MedicineNet, a website of U.S. Board Certified Physicians and Allied Health Professionals: www.medicinenet.com

Memorial Urology Associates, Houston, Texas: www.houston-urology.com/default.htm

National Institute on Aging, "Sexuality in Later Life": www.niapublications.org

National Parkinson's Foundation: www.parkinson.org

Period Life Tables: www.ssa.gov/

Prostate cancer statistics: prostate-help.org/castats.htm

Sexuality Information and Education Council of the U.S. (SIECUS): www.siecus.org

The American Heart Association: www.Americanheart.org

The American Society on Aging: www.asaging.org

The Arthritis Foundation: www.arthritis.org

The Male Reproductive System: www.betterhealth.vic.gov

Index

About the Authors

Leah Kliger, MHA, has had a 33-year career in health care as an educator, author, consultant, executive, and researcher. She is an assistant clinical professor in the Department of Health Services at the University of Washington, Seattle and co-founder of Women Beyond 50 LLC. In the 1970s, Leah spent three years running a Family Planning clinic and counseling young people about sexuality. In her early 50s, she realized that there was a deafening silence about sexuality in the aging woman, leading her to conclude that this topic needed to be brought out from under the covers. Leah is a frequent conference speaker and a writer. She's had a number of magazine articles published that delve into women's sexuality at mid life and beyond. In 2000, Leah authored a first-of-its-kind report, *Creating an Herbal Apothecary: A Guide for Physicians, Hospitals and Health Care Systems,* published by Health Care Communications, Inc. She contributed two chapters to *Integrating Complementary Medicine into Health Systems,* by Nancy Faass, editor, published by Aspen Publishing in 2001.

Leah graduated with a B.S. from Michigan State University, East Lansing, Michigan, and holds a Masters in health care administration from the University of Washington, Seattle. She and her husband, Phil, have been married for 12 years and live in Kirkland, Washington. As a wife, mother, step-mother, mother-in-law, grandmother, sister, aunt, and friend, she personally understands the impact of shifting sexuality on women's lives.

Deborah Nedelman, Ph.D., has had a 30-year career as a licensed clinical psychologist and maintained a private psychotherapy practice in Everett, Washington through 2004. She is a certified sex therapist and co-founder of Women Beyond 50 LLC. Deborah has talked with hundreds of women and couples over many years about sexual concerns. Several years ago she realized that as she had gotten older, so had her clients. They began asking, "What is normal for the older woman?" And there were few definitive answers. Her mission is now to ignite a global discussion about older women's sexuality.

Deborah graduated from Bryn Mawr College and holds a Ph.D. in clinical psychology from the University of Washington. In 1977, Dr. Nedelman co-authored *A Guide for Beginning Psychotherapists,* published by Cambridge University Press. This work has been translated into 10 languages and remained in print until 2002. She and her husband, Mel, have been married for 31 years and are the parents of two adult children.

Learn more about Leah and Deborah at www.womenbeyond50.com, or contact them at info@womenbeyond50.com.